10-MINUTE WORKOUTS FOR SENIORS 60+

Simple Illustrated Exercises Elderly of Any Level Can Do at Home to Drastically Improve Balance, Strength and Whole-Body Wellness | 4-Week Plan Included

Steve Donovan

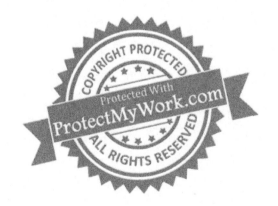

TABLE OF CONTENTS

INTRODUCTION

When you age, your body changes, and it can be hard to keep up with the demands of being a healthy senior. But this doesn't mean there's no hope of maintaining or improving your health as you age. Depending on how old you are and how physically active you were in your younger years, a wide range of exercises are available to help maintain your fitness level and improve strength, power, and balance. One thing that many seniors often overlook is their diet- when making adjustments to food choices (e.g. switching from car to walking, or walking to biking), exercise (e.g. moving from the couch to a regular exercise routine), and other lifestyle choices (e.g. quitting smoking, getting more sleep) it's easy to forget about maintaining a healthy diet that is packed with vitamins and nutrients that can help your body function better as you age.

Exercise is an important part of an overall lifestyle change for seniors as it helps them maintain the balance, strength and mobility of aging. Exercises can also:

In addition to the health benefits of exercise, you may experience a boost in your self-confidence, mood and energy levels. Working out can even help relieve stress and anxiety.

Many kinds of exercises can be done to help improve your physical health as you get older. The exercise you choose depends on your current fitness level and goal. For example, if walking is enough to get your heart rate up as part of an aerobic workout, then that's what you should do. On the other hand, you may want to try strength training if you need to improve your strength.

Almost everyone knows about cardio exercises such as running, bicycling and walking. Aerobic exercises get the heart rate up to the point where it's working hard enough that oxygen is being used efficiently by the muscles. Anaerobic exercise is different from aerobic exercise in that anaerobic workouts use oxygen at a high rate but are not efficient enough for the muscles to function optimally. Aerobic exercise uses oxygen all day, every day, and for long periods. This exercise helps maintain a healthy heart and helps build healthy bones because it keeps your muscles strong and flexible. Examples of aerobic exercises are walking, jogging, and biking.

Resistance training helps tone muscles. It can help improve muscle strength and power. Examples of resistance exercises include weight training and body weight exercises such as push-ups and squats. Resistance training is a great way to help maintain your strength level as you age because it helps build up your muscles. As we grow older, our muscles become weaker, so we must keep them strong by doing strength-training exercises every day.

Stretching is another exercise that improves flexibility and balance, which helps reduce the chances of falling and fracturing a bone. Stretching also boosts the range of motion in your joints. Flexibility can help you avoid injuries and recover from certain injuries that may have occurred because of falling.

Flexibility exercises include stretching and strength training exercises. Strength training exercises are designed to build up the strength in your muscles, which helps support healthy connective tissue (such as cartilage and tendons) in addition to helping you maintain a healthy weight. How often you need to stretch will depend on your age, overall health, fitness level, physical activity levels, the weather and other factors.

A common form of stretching is called flexibility training because it improves flexibility. Flexibility training is designed to improve your mobility and range of motion. While some people choose to stretch on their own, it's often recommended that you stretch with the help of a physical therapist or certified trainer who can help modify your stretches as needed to make them more effective.

Aerobic exercises such as walking, jogging, running, cycling and swimming are good choices for seniors looking to increase their heart rate and burn extra calories. These exercises will also help build endurance and improve your respiratory system so you can breathe better when engaged in daily activities. If you're just making changes in your exercise routine, start out slow and gradually build up your stamina over time.

Some seniors may want to include strength-training exercises in their daily workout routine. Strength training exercises are designed to help you build up your muscles, which can increase your strength and help you maintain a healthy weight. If you're looking for ways to improve your overall health by adding muscle strength, push-ups and pull-ups can be a great way to get started. These exercises strengthen the back, shoulders and arms and are easy on the joints by working against gravity instead of perpendicular muscle contractions.

THE IMPORTANCE OF EXERCISING FOR SENIORS

Many people who are older than 60 years old may have their health decline if they don't exercise. There are enough benefits from joining in with weight-bearing exercises, such as improving bone density, strengthening the heart and lungs, lowering blood pressure and cholesterol levels, slowing down cognitive decline and more. Seniors will be able to live for a longer time if they exercise because exercising will not only increase physical movement but it will also help mental stimulation.

No matter what your age is or how much you've been doing since before your twenties, there's no reason why you should be out of shape anymore. You can do it if you want to feel good, get in shape, and live a healthy life.

WHAT IS EXERCISE?

The best way to define exercise is by saying that it's a physical activity that you perform to help maintain or improve your health. Walking around your neighborhood or taking a walk at the park are great ways to exercise. Take note that there's nothing to stop you from exercising indoors if you prefer this fitness method over going outdoors. You don't have to go out of your way from time to time just because it's winter. You can walk around the house, make short runs around the block, and do sit-ups in your room; the important thing here is: moving your body.

WHAT IS WEIGHT-BEARING EXERCISE?

Weight-bearing exercises are those activities that involve the bones and muscles that make up your muscles. These activities can be done in a club, home or anywhere else where you can run around, jump and hop while performing physical activities like running, jumping or jumping rope. Running on a treadmill may not be as fun as a game of football with your friends, but it's still an important part of weight-bearing exercise for adults over 60.

EXERCISE IS GREAT FOR BOTH YOUR MENTAL AND PHYSICAL HEALTH

One of the ways that exercise can aid your mental health is by helping you cope with stress when you have it. For example, studies have shown that when seniors feel stressed, participating in a form of weight-bearing exercise will help them better handle the stress than if they don't do anything. So if you're having a stressful day, get out and go for a run or walk around the block. When you feel better after exercising, it's easier for your body to stop having so much cortisol (stress hormone).

Exercise is also very good for improving your mood. When your body releases endorphins in the brain, you feel like you're high even though no drugs are involved. These happy feelings from endorphins make you more likely to be happy and help you stay positive throughout the day. So even though you won't always feel like it, exercise is important to keep yourself healthy and strong.

THE IMPORTANCE OF EXERCISE FOR SENIORS

Since seniors are more likely to gain weight, exercise is even more important for them than for younger people. By participating in weight-bearing exercises, you can help yourself to be healthier and stronger. You won't worry about having problems doing ordinary things because your muscles will be strong and flexible enough to do anything that you need to do at any time. You cannot completely avoid gaining weight as you get older. Still, by exercising regularly and being healthy, you won't have a problem with it getting too bad.

BENEFITS OF EXERCISE FOR SENIORS

As you get older, the body loses muscle mass and agility. By participating in weight-bearing exercises, you can improve those things and help your body be as healthy as it can be. Some of the benefits that come from exercising include:

- Helps to prevent osteoporosis

- Helps to lessen back pain

- Helps to increase bone density

- Increases flexibility

- Improves cardiovascular fitness

- Reduces stress levels

Exercising is the most important thing you can do to live a long and healthy life. Suppose you want to be active and participate in physical activities as an adult. In that case, you have to get involved in weight-bearing exercise. In time, you won't have any problems with your muscles because they'll be strong and flexible enough to do everything you need.

HOW TO DEVELOP THE HABIT OF WORKING OUT

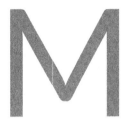any people have the misconception that exercising is a chore they must do. This problem can last for years, even decades. In this chapter, I will give tips to help you develop the habit of working out even when you don't want to do it right now. These tips have helped me become more disciplined and motivated to work out.

1. NEVER SKIP A WORKOUT.

This is the most difficult piece of advice on the list to follow; after all, the issue is getting into the mindset to exercise. But here's the thing: you can't get into a workout mindset without working out. The good news is that as you create exercise routines.

Plan two to four workouts per week and stick to it. There will be days when you don't feel like working out, but unless you're sick, force yourself to do so. You can cut your workout short or do something simple. Making fitness a habit is key to having an active life. It'll be a lot easier to stick to a regimen after that.

2. FIND SOMETHING YOU ENJOY DOING.

You're not going to have a nice time if you despise running but force yourself onto the treadmill. Finding an activity you enjoy is the key to getting into the appropriate mindset.

Running, elliptical use, cycling, studio courses, and other alternatives are available. Working out at home will become much easier once you have a favorite activity.

3. ESTABLISH GOALS AND KEEP A VISUAL RECORD OF YOUR PROGRESS.

If you don't feel like you're making any progress, you could find it difficult to motivate yourself to exercise. Nobody enjoys working for no pay, but you might be making more progress than you realize.

Setting defined goals and tracking your progress over time is the greatest method to overcome this issue.

For example, every treadmill run may feel the same, but if you track your workouts, you may see that your pace has grown or that you can run for longer periods. Numerous apps are available to help you track your workouts, or you may use a good old-fashioned notebook. And believe me when I say that development is satisfying and will have you returning for more!

4. LOOK FOR INSPIRATION

A picture is worth a thousand words and may also increase your motivation by 1,000 percent. So surround yourself with images that motivate you to be active if you need that extra push to head to workout at home. This could be photos of your favorite athlete, other people's progress, or photos of a dream location such as Mount Everest.

You can add a dose of visual motivation to your day by creating a Pinterest board, following your favorite athletes on Instagram, or cutting out photographs from fitness magazines. Your lifestyle change will be guided by this vision board.

5. REMIND YOURSELF WHY YOU'RE LIVING AN ACTIVE LIFE

Every time you work out, remind yourself why you joined the club in the first place. Consider how happy you'll be when you achieve your objectives. You're investing time and work that will pay off later, and it will all be worthwhile.

Even if working out appears a nuisance, adopting a grateful mindset and appreciating your body's ability to move may make each sweat session more enjoyable. Get to work!

HOW SENIORS CAN GET STARTED

f you are interested in starting a workout plan but have hesitations or don't know where to start, there's no better time than now.

Most of your retirement years will be spent in the comfort of your home, and you can use that time to get fit and healthy! Start with basic movements like squats, push-ups, sit-ups, and lunges. Next, you'll tone muscles and make moves like getting up from a seated position easier and boosting your balance. Make sure not to overwork yourself, though! Just set a goal for 5 more minutes of exercise each day until you're up to 30 minutes.

Limited mobility or physical restrictions may make certain types of exercise inadvisable. Talk to your doctor about the best exercises for you.

Start slowly to avoid injury and increase the amount of time spent being physical as you feel more comfortable. Don't hesitate to ask your doctor if you have questions or concerns.

Aerobic exercises are any activity that uses large muscle groups, which increases your heart pumping and respiration rate. Low-impact exercises like walking, swimming, and cycling are great choices that negatively impact the joints.

The NIA recommends 150 minutes a week of moderate aerobic activity or 75 minutes a week of vigorous aerobic exercise, or an equivalent combination of moderate and vigorous activity.

Your workout should be varied and use all the muscles in your body. If you're just starting out, focus on building your endurance before attempting more advanced exercises like running and swimming.

Focus on reducing stress as much as possible while doing any physical activity. Stress increases cortisol in our bodies, leading to loss of muscle mass and function, low energy levels, lower metabolism and weight gain.

Try to clear your mind and get rid of all anxious thoughts. Do this by listening to music or other soothing sounds but avoid stressful television shows and conversations with demanding people.

In addition to stress reduction, yoga and meditation have been shown to have several other health benefits, including improved lung capacity, stronger immune system and better breathing.

Some people feel overwhelmed by the thought of starting a new workout routine so consider a beginner's fitness class such as Tai Chi or Aqua Fit for your first attempt at exercise. You can find classes taught by an instructor at the YMCA or community center.

The first step is important because failure helps you understand that you can achieve what you set out to do. Then you'll take that information and apply it to other workouts.

Start with something simple like walking for a few minutes a day. Keeping a record of your progress will go a long way toward motivating you to stick with physical activity throughout your life. You can keep track of your progress by fitness journaling, which is recording your workout data, as well as the reasons why you exercised and how they made you feel.

Remember that there is no one-size-fits-all workout program. Try different exercises, find ones that are right for you and make sure the routine is enjoyable!

HOW TO APPROACH THE WORKOUT

The benefits of warming up are astounding. In fact, it's no exaggeration to say that warming up is one of the keys to enjoying a healthy life.

Warming up can help you prevent muscle injuries, relieve joint pain, and maintain performance throughout your workouts. If you're not careful, however, heart-arresting conditions such as heart attack or stroke are more likely to occur if you don't warm up properly.

Your body's circulation system isn't functioning properly when you're cold. But if you start with a good warm-up, you'll get the circulation moving, and it will continue to work properly throughout your day.

When you do a warm-up exercise correctly, every joint, muscle group and organ benefits from the process. This sets the stage for your entire day's workout to be productive and enjoyable.

For example, in the morning, I usually do jogging for about 20 minutes on the treadmill before I go out of bed at 8:30 am. This is one example of how a warm-up can help me perform better throughout the day. I feel strong and confident knowing that I got my blood flowing before facing the rest of my workouts, which can be very demanding.

On the other hand, if you don't warm up properly, your workout can easily become a fiasco and a complete waste of your time. The fat-burning effects of an exercise session will decrease, along with strength-building power. Another downside is that you're more apt to experience muscle injury or joint pain at some point.

Your body's biggest enemy right after sleep is your muscles' decreased circulation flow. Warming up opens your body's circulatory flow and prepares it for efficient digestion and effective cleansing.

The importance of warming up is straightforward, but convincing yourself that it's so worth the investment might be difficult. If you feel that a warm-up exercise is too hard, you can always choose an easier one that will give you the same benefits. And if you still feel that warming up isn't worth it, skip the workout and make up for it tomorrow (or whenever your schedule permits).

As mentioned above, warming up prepares your body for what's ahead. It also allows muscle groups to get acquainted with each other so they can interact more thoroughly throughout the entire workout.

Warming up also reduces muscle strain from exercises involving large muscles like your legs and arms. It also sets your body at ease to relax your breathing and relieve stress during a workout.

Warming up provides joint mobility, which allows you to perform the exercises more easily and lets you burn more calories while improving flexibility in the joints.

Warming up keeps your metabolism active, speeding up fat burning and boosting energy levels. It also increases your body's ability to absorb nutrients from food, enhancing recovery and increasing energy levels throughout the day.

Warming up also increases blood flow around nerves, preventing muscle pulls, strains or cramps.

In short, warming up makes your workout more effective and efficient, allowing you to enjoy positive benefits throughout the day.

Are you convinced yet?

DYNAMIC STRETCHES AND STATIC STRETCHES

n the world of sports, dynamic stretches are becoming more and more popular compared to static stretching. It's a common misconception that static stretching is better for warming up. Still, the truth is: that dynamic stretches have so many benefits over static stretches that it's no wonder they're trending.

In this part, we'll be discussing why you should choose dynamic stretches over static stretches for warming up.

THE BENEFITS OF DYNAMIC STRETCHING

There are a few specific benefits that dynamic stretching has over static stretching. When a muscle is warmed up, it can get stiff and hard to move. When this happens, static stretching will help loosen up the muscle and make it more pliable. However, there are many drawbacks to static stretching for warming up. Static stretches can be tedious because you must keep changing angles and positions throughout the routine. Not only is this counterproductive, but it can cause serious harm.

Dynamic stretching can greatly decrease the time it takes to warm up muscles. Your muscles will be gently stretched instead of being held under extreme tension by having to focus on moving at the right angle and position.

This allows your muscles to relax, resulting in enhanced performance and less injury. It also means more flexibility throughout your workout.

THE BENEFITS OF DYNAMIC STRETCHING WHILE WORKING OUT

There are a couple benefits dynamic stretching has while working out that static stretching doesn't provide. To start, dynamic stretches will help relieve stiffness and soreness that often feel after a workout session. The quick movements of dynamic stretches will help increase blood circulation, which will bring fresh oxygen and nutrients to your muscles.

Your body will recover faster and more efficiently after every session. Dynamic stretching also helps improve coordination, balance, and awareness of your body position. This way, your workouts will be more effective and efficient. If you're looking to improve performance in your home or on the field at work, then dynamic stretching is a must!

As you can see from this part, dynamic stretches have plenty of benefits over static stretching. By using dynamic stretches before static stretches, you can boost your body's performance in your house while also getting rid of any stiffness you may have.

Suppose you want to gain better flexibility, improve joint mobility, or just have a powerful workout. In that case, I urge you to give dynamic stretching a try!

WARMING-UP EXERCISES

1. Shoulder Rolls

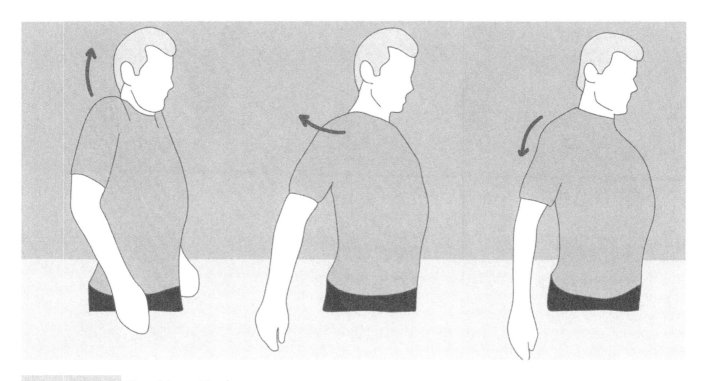

Targeted Area: Shoulders, Neck

Difficulty: Easy

Directions:

- Stand with legs shoulder-width apart.

- Start the rotation by raising both shoulders toward the ears for 3 seconds.

- At this point, imagine bringing the shoulders behind you as much as possible while retracting the shoulder blades. Hold the position for 3 seconds

- Now, actively push the shoulders down for 3 seconds.

- The final position of the sequence is with shoulders pushed forward and chest in toward the spine. Hold this position for another 3 seconds.

- Repeat the cycle 2 more times.

2. Leg Swings

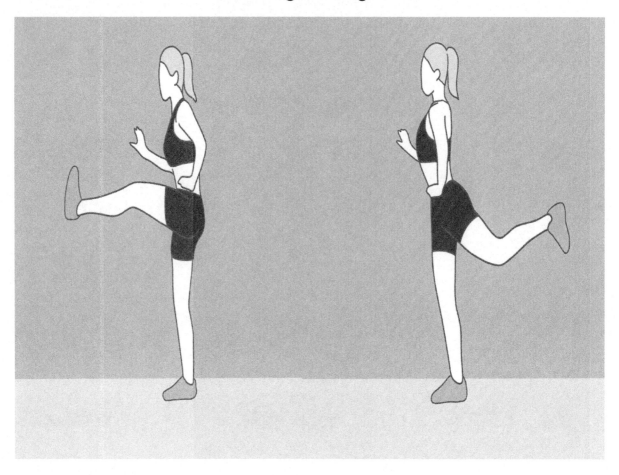

Targeted Area: Glutes, Hamstrings, Quads

Difficulty: Medium

Directions:

- Place your palm flat against a wall or grab the back of a table or chair for better stability

- As if you're kicking a ball, with the leg slightly bent, swing your right leg forward. Kick as high as you can without losing balance or twisting your torso.

- The leg should then be swung back behind you. You won't be able to go back as far as you'd like.

- Repeat 10–15 times more, then do the same for the other leg.

3. Ankle Circles

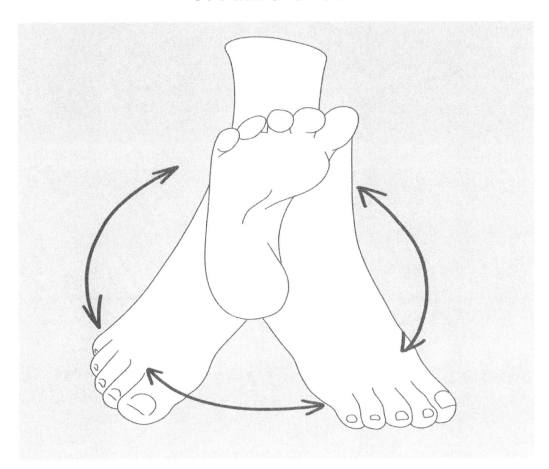

Targeted Area: Ankle

Difficulty: Easy

Directions:

Directions:

- Sit on a chair with your back straight.

- Hold yourself to the chair's seat with both hands for better stability.

- Rotate your right foot as if you were painting a circle in the air.

- Switch to the opposing foot after 10 to 20 complete ankle rotations.

4. Hamstring Stretch

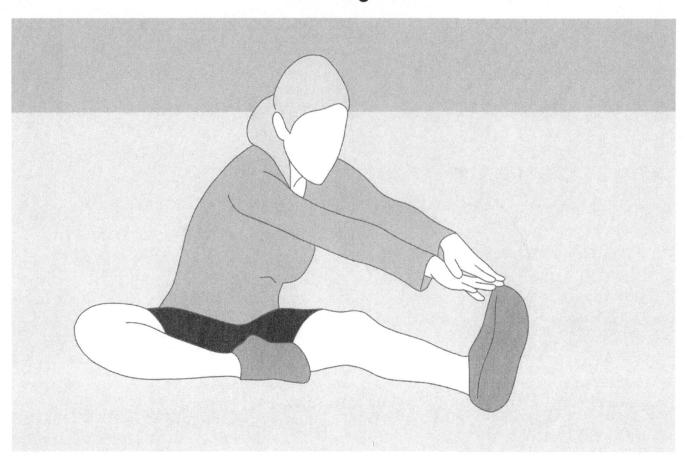

Targeted Area: Hamstrings, Calves

Difficulty: Medium

Directions:

- Sit on a mat with your left leg stretched in front of you

- Rest the heel of your right foot on your left thigh.

- Stretch both arms toward the left leg and aim to grab the foot

- Pull the foot toward you for a deeper stretch

- Hold this position for 30 seconds.

- Repeat the exercise for the other leg.

5. Shin Stretch

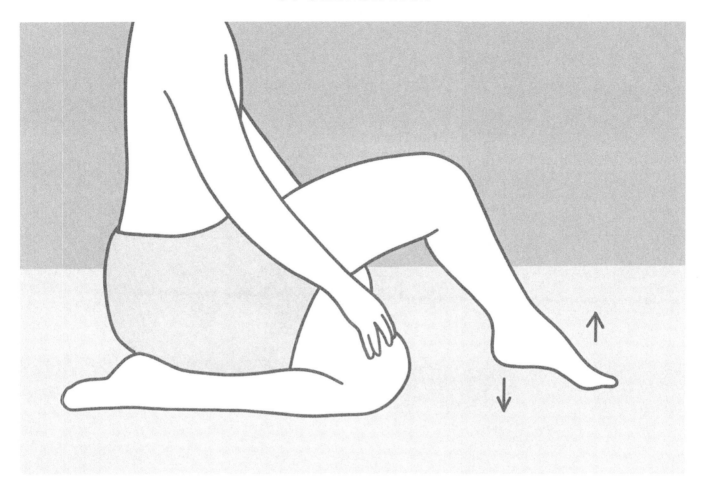

Targeted Area: Ankle, Calf

Difficulty: Easy

Directions:

- Sit on your right leg, with the heel touching the glutes.

- As shown in the figure, raise the heel of the left leg off the floor and put the weight on the toes. You should focus on stretching the calf.

- Hold the stretch for 5 seconds, then bring the heel back on the floor.

- Repeat the exercise 10 times total, then do the same for the other side.

6. Hip Lifts

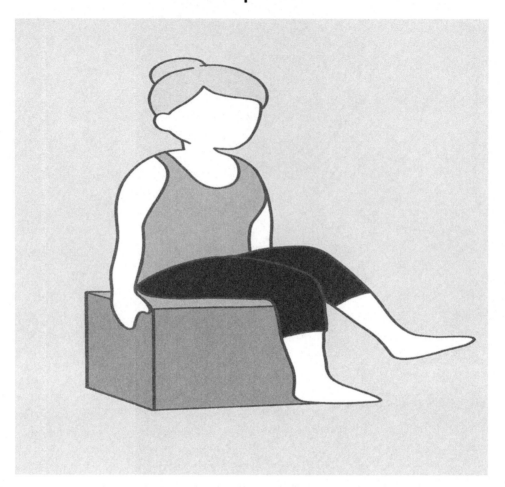

Targeted Area: Quads

Difficulty: Easy

Directions:

- Sit on a chair with your back straight.

- Hold to the chair's seat for better stability

- Raise your right knee and hip off the chair as high as possible.

- Hold it for 3-5 seconds.

- Do the same for the other leg.

- Repeat the exercise 5 times per side.

7. Waist Circles

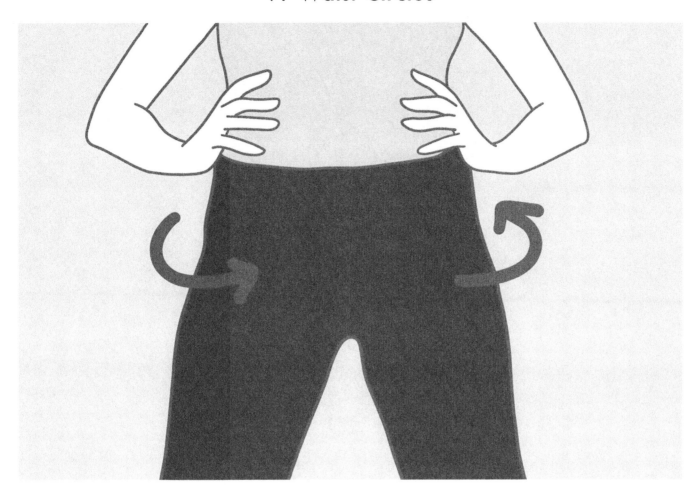

Targeted Area: Hips, Lower back

Difficulty: Easy

Directions:

- Stand with legs shoulder-width apart, straight back and chin facing in front of you.

- Rest both hands on your waist

- Starting slowly, rotate your hips to the left (counterclockwise) aiming for a 360° movement. Imagine to be painting a big circle on the ground with your waist.

- Repeat the movement for 5 big cirles.

- Do the same movement clockwise for 5 big circles.

8. Quad Stretch

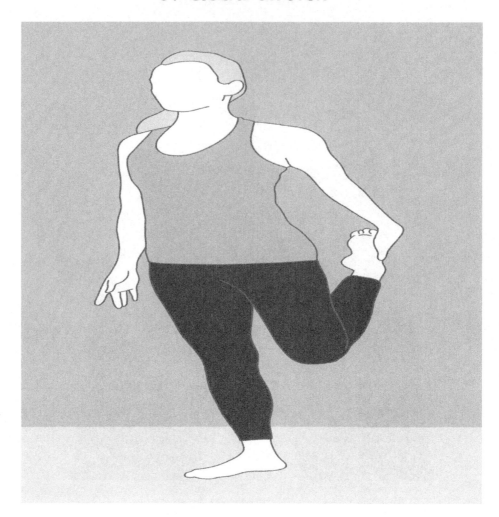

Targeted Area: Hips, Quads

Difficulty: Easy

Directions:

- Stand with legs shoulder-width apart.

- Lift your left foot behind you and grab it with your left hand, shifting the body weight to your right leg.

- Slowly pull your foot up to your bottom as much as needed to feel a nice stretch in the quad. If your knee hurts, stop the exercise.

- Hold the position for around 30 seconds.

- Repeat the exercise for the other leg.

9. Hip Rollover

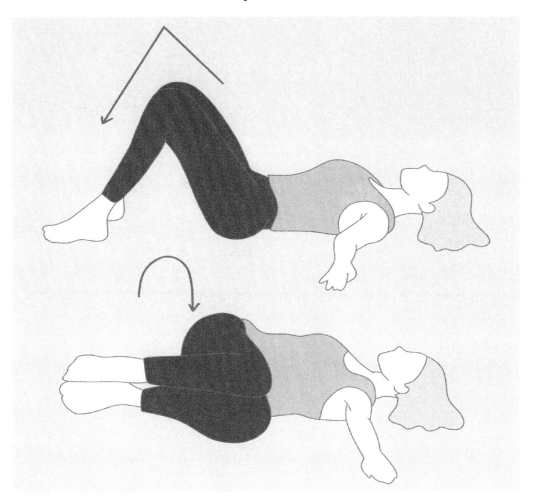

Targeted Area: Lower back, Upper back, Shoulders, Glutes

Difficulty: Hard

Directions:

- Lie on a mat with your knees forming an angle as in the first picture and arms straight pointing on the sides.

- Inhale deeply. As you exhale, slowly drop both knees to the left, trying to stretch the muscles on the right side. During this movement, exhale slowly and focus on the stretch.

- Try to stay in this position for at least 5 seconds

- Repeat the exercise on the other side for a total of 3 times per side.

10-MINUTE WORKOUT ROUTINES

SITTING WORKOUT

1. Knee Extensions

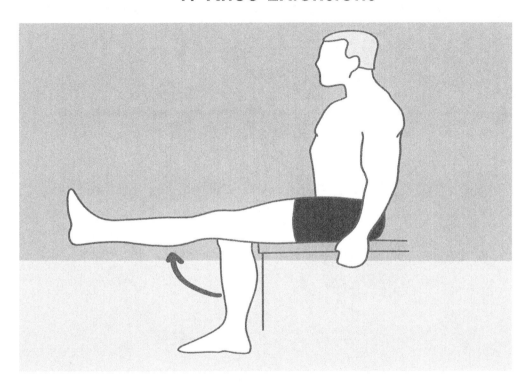

Sets x Repetitions: 10x5"

Muscles targeted: Quads

Equipment needed: Chair

Directions:

- Sit on a chair with your back straight while holding to the chair's seat for better stability,

- Raise your left leg in front of you and keep it straight, while focusing on contracting the quadricep.

- Hold this position for 5 seconds. Do the same for the other leg for a total of 10 sets per leg.

2. Pillow Squeeze

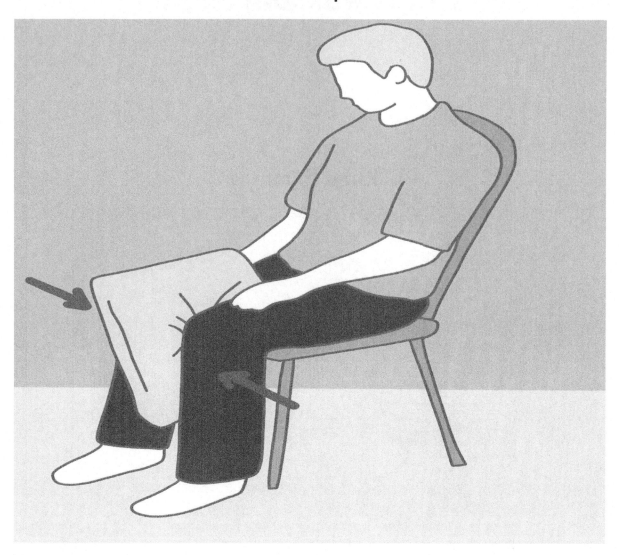

Sets x Repetitions: 12x3"

Muscles targeted: Adductors

Equipment needed: Chair, Pillow

Directions:

- Sit on a chair with your back straight and put a pillow between the knees.

- Contract your inner thigh muscles to squeeze the pillow as hard as you can.

- Squeeze for 3 seconds and then relax.

- Repeat the exercise 12 times total.

3. Clamshells

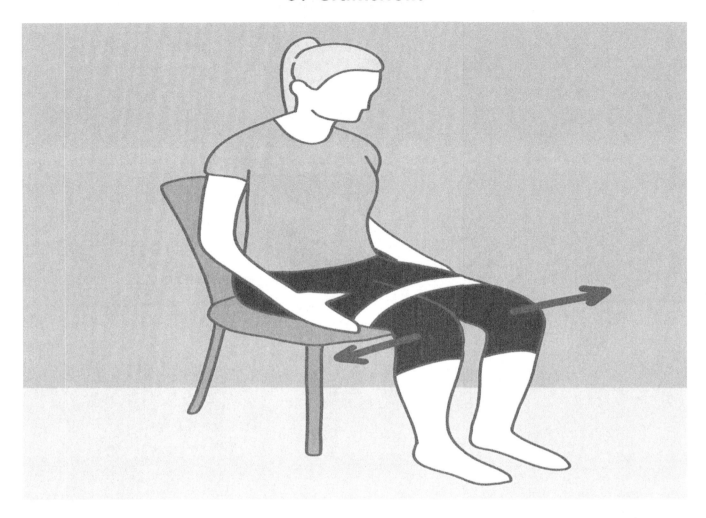

Sets x Repetitions: 12x3"

Muscles targeted: Abductors

Equipment needed: Chair, Resistance band

Directions:

- Sit on a chair with your back straight and a resistance band around your legs (a few inches above the knees)

- Push the knees away from each other, opening as much as you can.

- Hold the position for 3 seconds.

- Repeat the exercise 12 times in total.

4. Marching

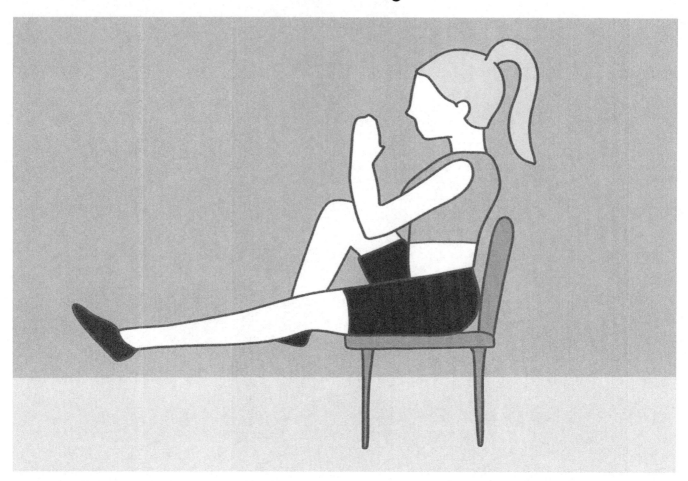

Sets x Repetitions: 2x30"

Muscles targeted: Legs

Equipment needed: Chair

Directions:

- Sit on a chair with your back straight with either your hands on the seat or as in the figure.

- Start marching with your legs, slowly alternating each other. You want to raise your knees as high as possible and straighten your leg completely in front of you. U

- Keep going for about 30 seconds total.

- Rest 30 seconds and repeat one more time.

5. Chair Squats

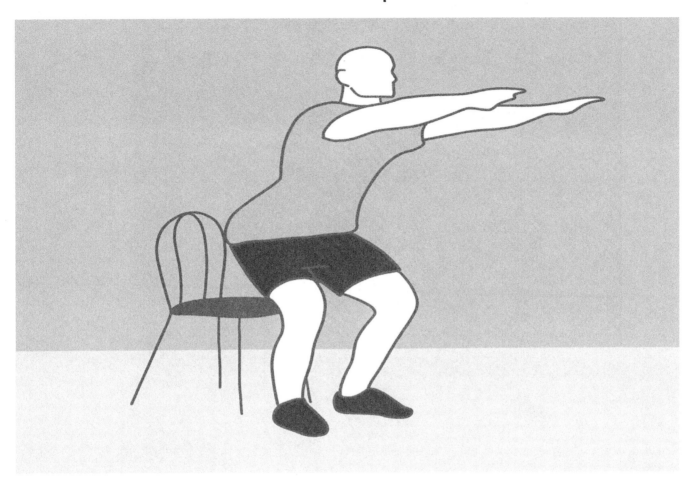

Sets x Repetitions: 3x8

Muscles targeted: Legs, Glutes

Equipment needed: Chair

Directions:

- Stand straight with legs shoulder-width apart (feet slightly pointing outwards) and a chair placed right behind you.

- Engage your abs and slowly start to sit back. Make sure to keep your chest up, abs engaged and back straight.

- Once your bottom touch the chair's seat, stand back up by pushing through the heels of your feet.

- Repeat the movement for 8 times total. Rest for 1 minute, then repeat two more times.

1. Side Raises

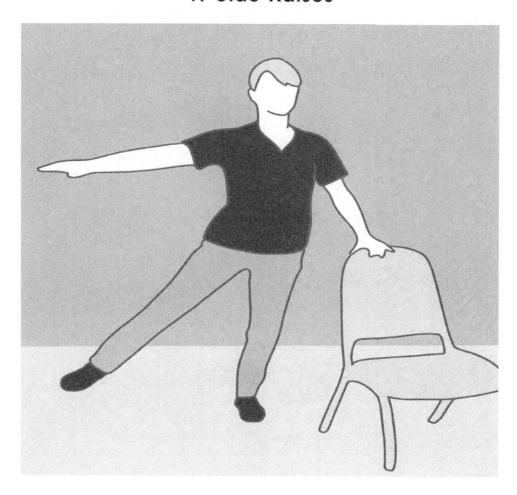

Sets x Repetitions: 5x10"

Muscles targeted: Abs, Legs, Shoulders

Equipment needed: Chair

Directions:

- Stand next to a chair and place your left hand on the backrest. If you think you can, try without the chair support.

- Raise your right arm and right leg simultaneously outward.

- Hold the position for 10 seconds and return to the starting position.

- Repeat the exercise 5 times and then do the same on the other side.

2. Weight Shifting

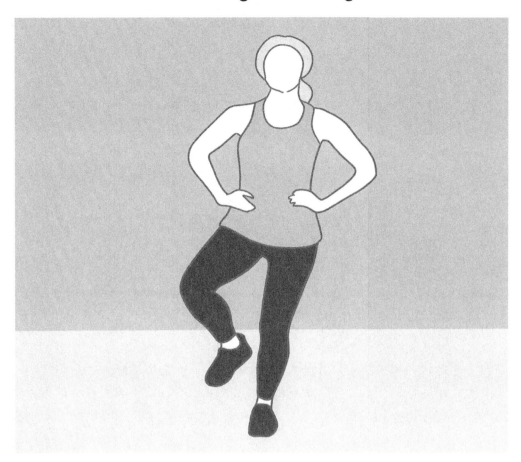

Sets x Repetitions: 5x15"

Muscles targeted: Abs, Quads

Equipment needed: None

Directions:

- Place both hands on your waist.

- Shift your body weight to your left leg and lift your right leg as high as possible.

- Hold the position for 15 seconds.

- Do the same on the other leg and repeat the exercise for a total of 5 times per leg.

3. Flamingo Stand

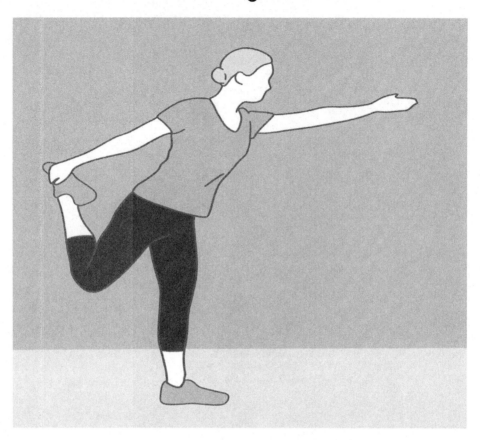

Sets x Repetitions: 2x30"

Muscles targeted: Abs, Quads

Equipment needed: None

Directions:

- Stand with legs shoulder-width apart.

- Lift your right foot behind you and grab it with your right hand, shifting the body weight to your left leg.

- Slowly pull your foot up to your bottom as much as needed to feel a nice stretch in the quad. If your knee hurts, stop the exercise.

- Raise your left arm in front of you and bend the torso outward until you feel your balance is getting unstable. Hold the position for around 30 seconds. Then, do the same for the other leg for a total of two sets per leg.

4. Side Leg Raises

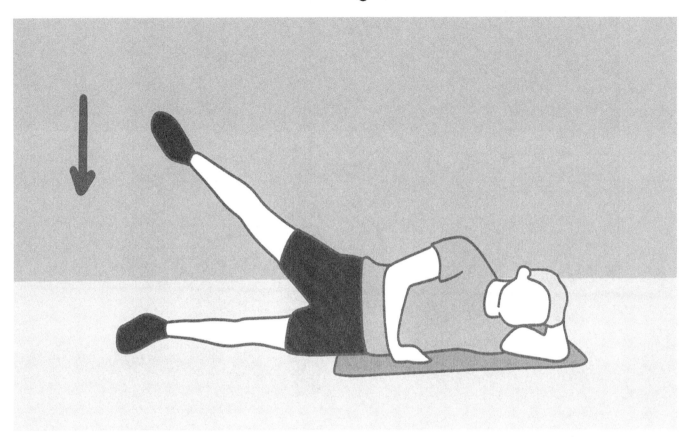

Sets x Repetitions: 10x3"

Muscles targeted: Abductors, Glutes

Equipment needed: Mat

Directions:

- Lie on your left side on a mat.

- Rest your head on your left arm.

- Rest the palm of your right hand on the mat for better stability.

- Raise your leg sideways as far as you can and hold the position for 3 seconds.

- Return to the starting position.

- Repeat the movement 10 times and then switch sides.

5. Tree Pose

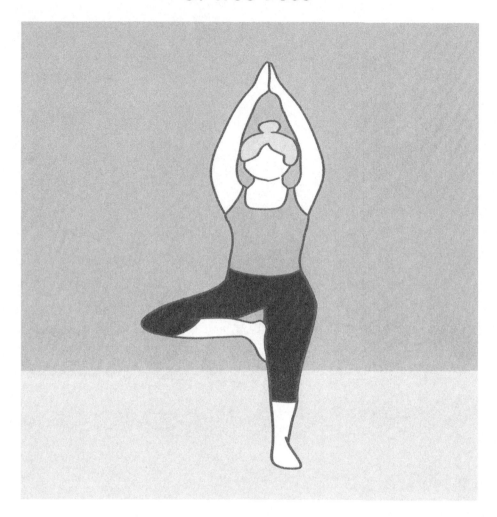

Sets x Repetitions: 2x30"

Muscles targeted: Abs, Legs

Equipment needed: None

Directions:

- Stand and place the sole of your right foot over the knee of your left leg, forming a 90° angle.

- Raise both arms above your head and press your hands together.

- Hold this position for 30 seconds and then switch legs.

- Repeat for a total of two times per side.

6. Step-Up

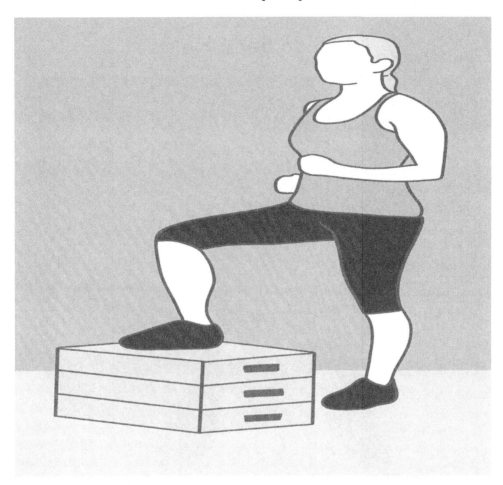

Sets x Repetitions: 1x30

Muscles targeted: Legs

Equipment needed: Box

Directions:

- Rest the sole of your right foot on a box. The box should be tall enough so that your knee forms a 90° angle when you rest your foot on it.

- Put your right foot on the box and quickly return to starting position.

- Use momentum to switch sides as quickly as you can and put your left foot on the box.

- Repeat the movement for a total of 30 steps per side.

1. Side Bend Holds

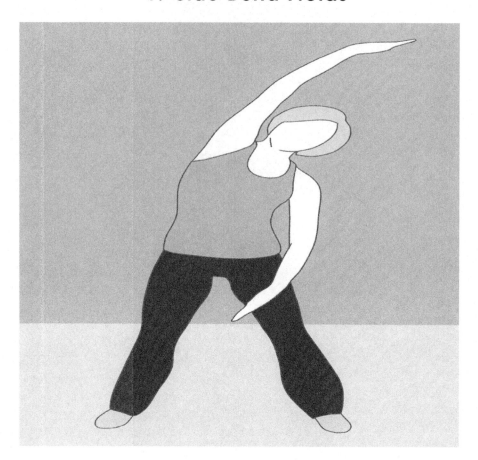

Sets x Repetitions: 4x10"

Muscles targeted: Abs, Lats

Equipment needed: None

Directions:

- Stand with legs open wide.

- Extend your right arm over your head. At the same time, lean your torso to the left side.

- Hold this position for 10 seconds.

- Do the same for the other side. Repeat 3 more times for each side.

2. Knee Raises

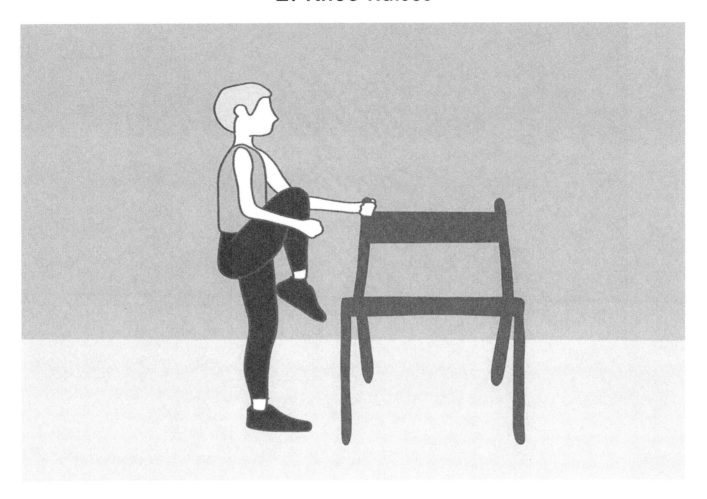

Sets x Repetitions: 3x20"

Muscles targeted: Glutes, Lower back

Equipment needed: None

Directions:

- Stand in front of a chair and grab the knee of your right leg with your right hand while holding onto the chair's back with the left hand for better stability

- Shift your body weight to your left leg.

- Pull the right knee as close to the chest as possible.

- Hold the position for 20 seconds and then repeat the exercise for the other leg.

3. Wall Snow Angel

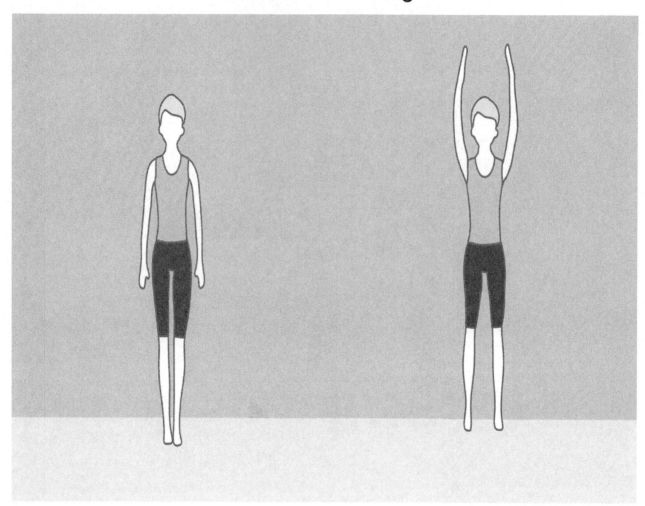

Sets x Repetitions: 1x8

Muscles targeted: Back, Shoulders

Equipment needed: None

Directions:

- Stand 15–20 cm (6–8 inches) from a wall. Lean against the wall with your bottom, back, shoulders, and head. Your hands will be touching your hips. By actively pushing your belly button toward your back, try to start with a neutral spine.

- As if drawing a big circle, move your arms straight up until they are over your head, as in the second figure. Always aim for the backs of your hands to never get off the wall during the movement.

- Slowly return to starting position. Repeat the exercise 8 times total.

4. Walking Heel-to-Toe

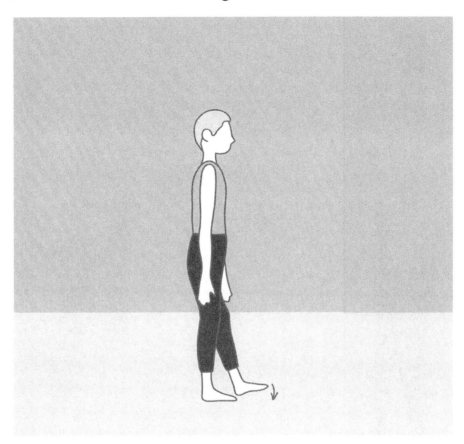

Sets x Repetitions: 2x60"

Muscles targeted: Abs, Ankles, Calves

Equipment needed: None

Directions:

- Stand with both your arms raised outward at shoulder level for better stability.

- Place your right foot in front of your left foot, with the heel of your right foot touching the toes of your left foot.

- Shift your weight on your heel as you put your left foot in front of your right.

- Now shift your weight to your toes.

- Repeat the steps with your left foot.

- Walk back and forth for a total of 60 seconds. Rest 30 seconds and then repeat one more time.

5. Knee Lift With Medicine Ball

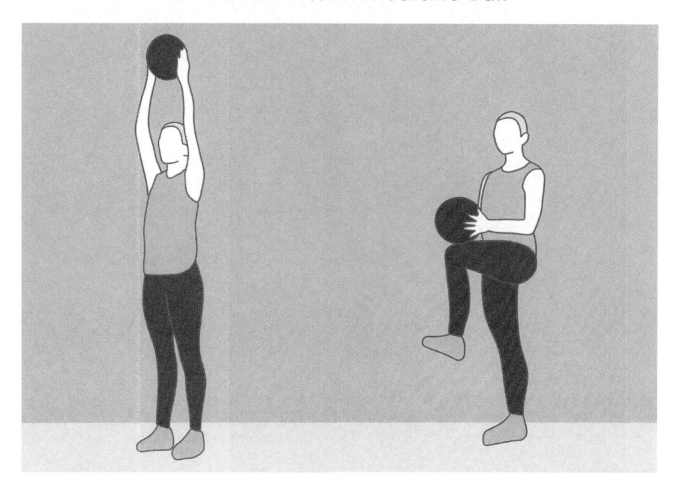

Sets x Repetitions: 2x10

Muscles targeted: Abs, Legs

Equipment needed: Medicine ball/Water bottle

Directions:

- Stand with your back straight and hold a medicine ball over your head. If you don't have it, use a weight or a 150oz water bottle.

- Raise the left knee to waist level while lowering both arms, bringing the weight or ball to the knee.

- Return the ball to its original position and lower the leg.

- Repeat the movement 9 more times.

- Do the same for the other side and repeat the process one more time.

1. Abdominal Bracing

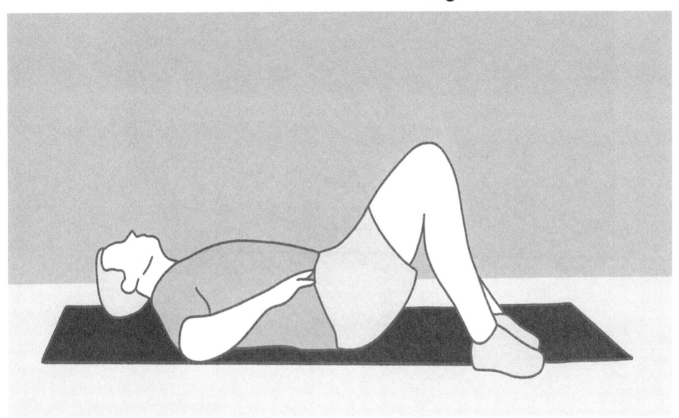

Sets x Repetitions: 2x45"

Muscles targeted: Abs

Equipment needed: Mat

Directions:

- Lie down on a mat with your knees slightly bent.

- Pull your belly button closer to your spine.

- Your abdominal muscles should tighten, assisting you in maintaining a great, straight posture.

- Remember to breathe normally and concentrate on keeping your belly button pulled in for 45 seconds.

- Repeat the exercise one more time.

2. Seated Knee Lifts

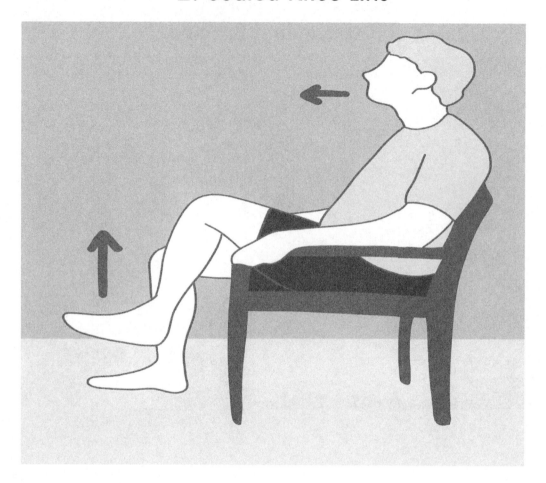

Sets x Repetitions: 5x5"

Muscles targeted: Abs

Equipment needed: Chair

Directions:

Sit on a chair with your back straight.

Hold to the chair's seat for better stability

Raise your left knee and hip off the chair as high as possible.

Hold it for 3-5 seconds.

Do the same for the other leg.

Repeat the exercise 5 times per side.

3. Seated Side Bends

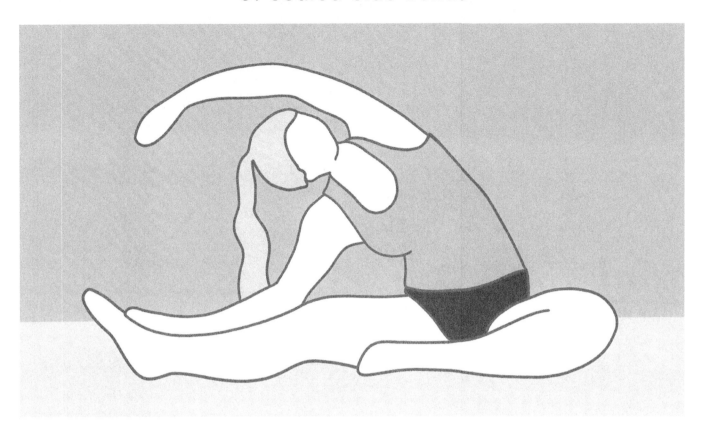

Sets x Repetitions: 2x10

Muscles targeted: Core, Lats

Equipment needed: Mat

Directions:

- Sit on a mat and extend your right leg outward.

- Bring the sole of your left foot a few inches above your right knee.

- With your right hand, try to grab the right foot.

- At this point, extend your left arm ìabove your head and aim to reach as close as possible to the right foot while stretching your torso at the same time. Hold the stretched position for 2 seconds.

- While keeping the right hand on the foot, bring your back and left arm back to starting position.

- Repeat the movement 10 times total. Rest 30 seconds, then repeat one more time.

- Do the same on the other side.

4. Dead Bug

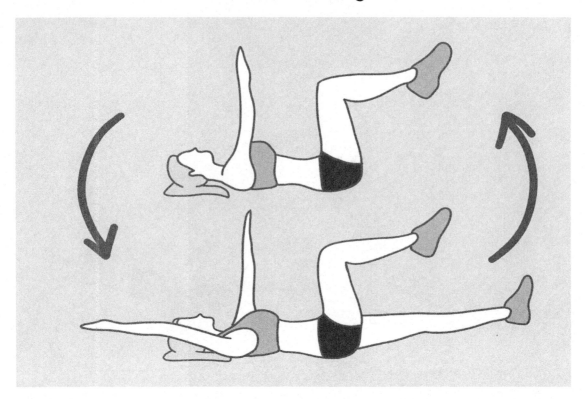

Sets x Repetitions: 2x10

Muscles targeted: Abs, Arms, Legs

Equipment needed: Mat

Directions:

- Lie down on a mat and raise both legs, forming a 90° angle.

- Raise both arms above your chest.

- Extend your left leg forward and bring your right arm to your right ear (straight).

- At this point, do the same movement on the opposite side while returning to starting position with the right arm and left leg. This alternating movement should be smooth.

- Repeat the exercise 10 times on each side. Rest 30 seconds, then repeat one more time.

P.S: The exercise done for both sides counts as 1 rep.

5. Glute Bridge

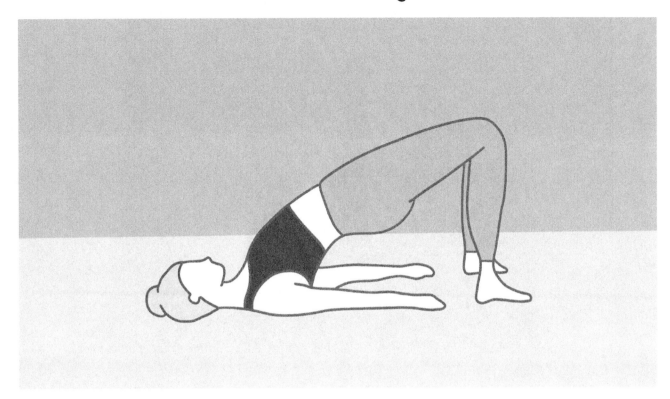

Sets x Repetitions: 5x15"

Muscles targeted: Glutes

Equipment needed: Mat

Directions:

- Lie down on a mat with your knees slightly bent, forming a 90° angle and your arms straight next to the body.

- Raise your bottom and hips off the floor by pushing through the heels as much as possible while maintaining a perfect balance.

- Hold this position for 15 seconds, then return to starting position.

- Repeat the movement 5 times total.

6. Side Leg Lift

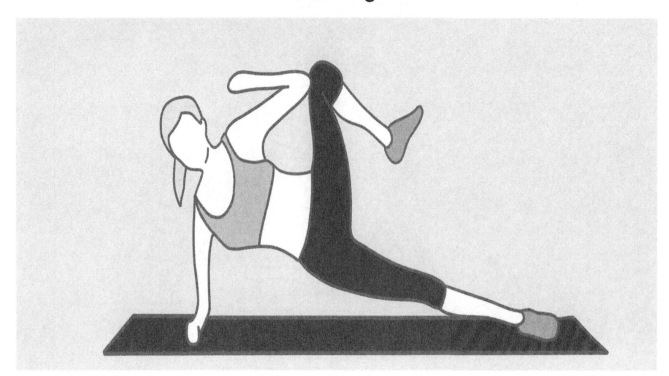

Sets x Repetitions: 2x5

Muscles targeted: Core

Equipment needed: Mat

Directions:

- Lie on your right side on a mat.

- Place your right arm at shoulder level as in the figure above and raise your body off the floor by pushing through the forearm.

- When you have found your balance, raise your left leg sideways until the knee touches your left elbow and return to the starting position.

- Repeat the movement 5 times and then switch sides.

- Rest 30 seconds and then repeat one more time

P.S: This is an advanced exercise. Feel free to skip it if it's too much for your current level.

7. Bird Dog

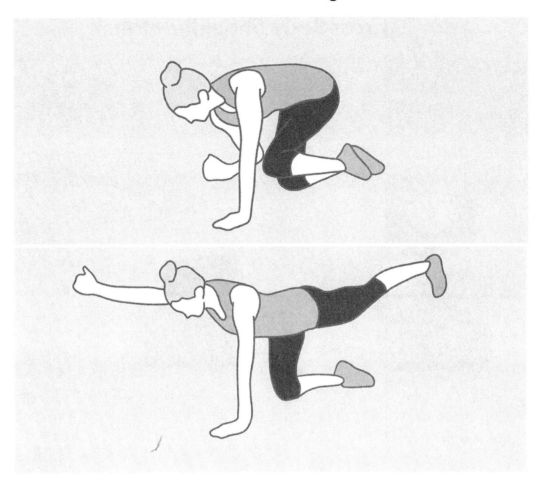

Sets x Repetitions: 2x8

Muscles targeted: Abs, Legs, Shoulders

Equipment needed: Mat

Directions:

- Start by getting on all fours. Then, simultaneously, bring the right elbow and left knee to each other until they touch.

- At this point, extend both in the opposite direction as in the figure above.

- Using the momentum, repeat the movement 7 more times.

- Do the same on the other side.

- Rest 30 seconds, then repeat the exercise one more time.

1. Cross-Body Shoulder Stretch

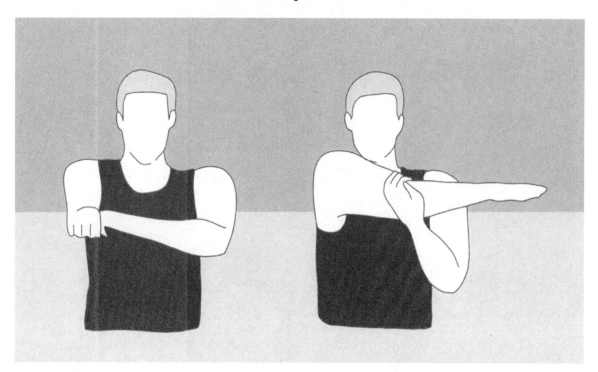

Sets x Repetitions: 2x20"

Muscles targeted: Shoulders, Upper back

Equipment needed: None

Directions:

- Stand with legs shoulder-width apart.

- Raise your right arm in front of you.

- Grab your right elbow with the left arm and pull it toward your left shoulder as much as you can (as in the figure).

- Hold this position for about 20 seconds.

- Do the same for the opposite side.

- Repeat the exercise for both sides one more time.

2. Neck and Trap Stretch

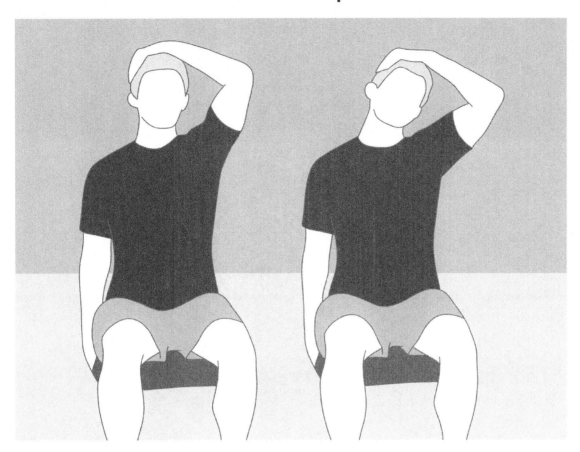

Sets x Repetitions: 1x30

Muscles targeted: Neck, Traps

Equipment needed: None/Chair

Directions:

- Sit on a chair with your back straight. You can also perform the exercise standing up.

- Grab the right side of your head with your left hand.

- Pull your head gently toward the left shoulder until you feel a mild stretch on your right side.

- Hold this position for 30 seconds.

- Repeat the exercise for the other side.

3. Chest Stretch

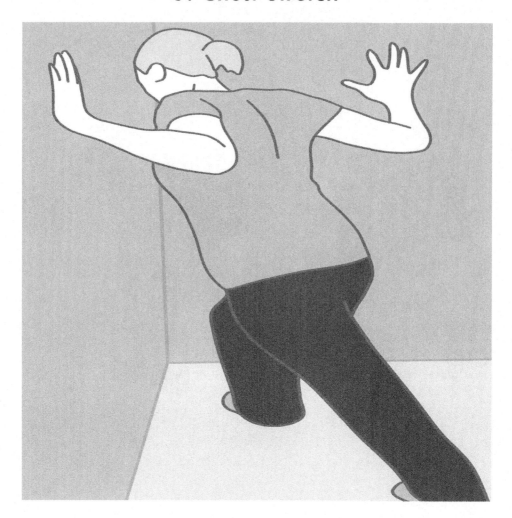

Sets x Repetitions: 2x30"

Muscles targeted: Chest, Shoulders

Equipment needed: None

Directions:

- Look for an angle in your room or house and place your palms on the sides of the walls

- Place one leg slightly bent in front of you while the other is straight behind you.

- Push through your palms so that your upper body moves forward until you feel a stretch in your chest and shoulders.

- Hold the stretch for 30 seconds. Rest for 20 seconds, then repeat one more time.

4. Overhead Reach

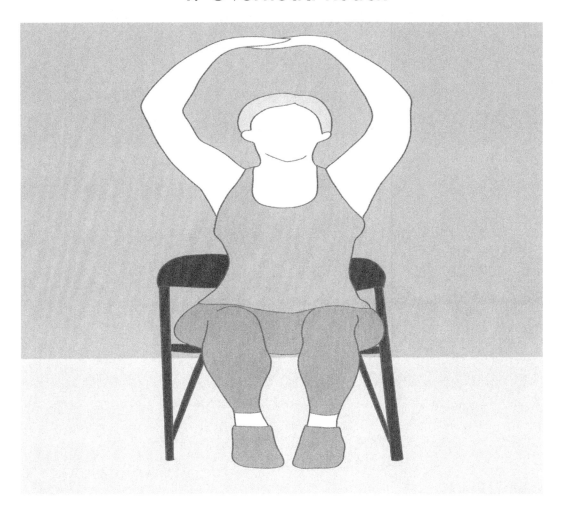

Sets x Repetitions: 2x20"

Muscles targeted: Arms, Shoulders, Upper back

Equipment needed: Chair

Directions:

- Raise your arms above your head and interlace your fingers, palms facing up.

- Stretch your arms toward the ceiling as much as possible.

- For a better stretch, think of stretching the right shoulder toward the ceiling as much as possible.

- Hold this position for 20 seconds. Repeat one more time.

5. Butterfly Stretch

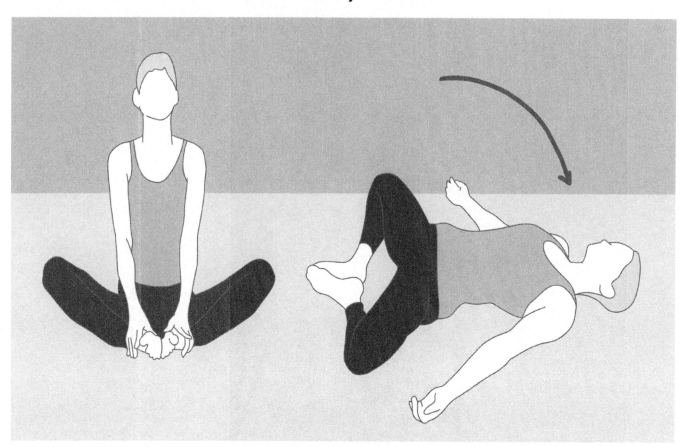

Sets x Repetitions: 2x40"

Muscles targeted: Hips, Inner thighs

Equipment needed: Mat

Directions:

- Sit on a mat.

- Press the heels of your feet toward each other and try to bring them close to your body as much as possible.

- While keeping your hands on the ankles, lie down once again.

- You can either actively push your feet toward your body or relax your arms as in the second picture.

- Hold this position for 40 seconds. Repeat one more time.

6. DownwarD-Facing Dog

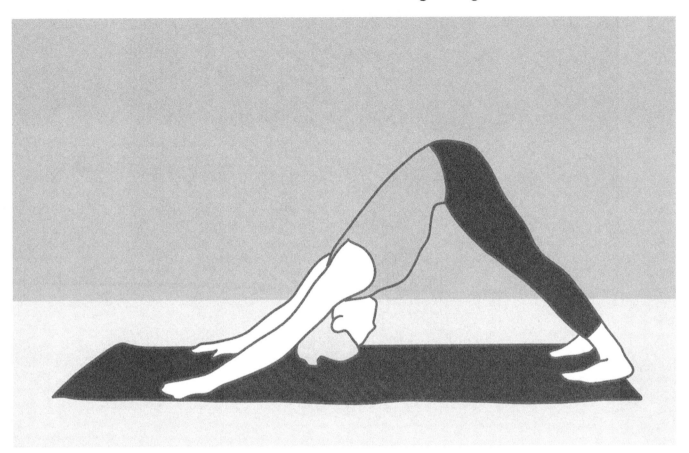

Sets x Repetitions: 3x20"

Muscles targeted: Abs, Legs, SHoulders

Equipment needed: Mat

Directions:

- Begin by resting on all fours on a mat, with both hands and feet placed farther from the body than you would normally.

- Raise your pelvis while resting your feet and palms on the floor.

- Contract your abs and bring your chin toward your lower body, maintaining a neutral curvature in your back and legs straight.

- Hold this position for 20 seconds.

- Rest for 20 seconds, then repeat the movement two more times.

7. Cobra

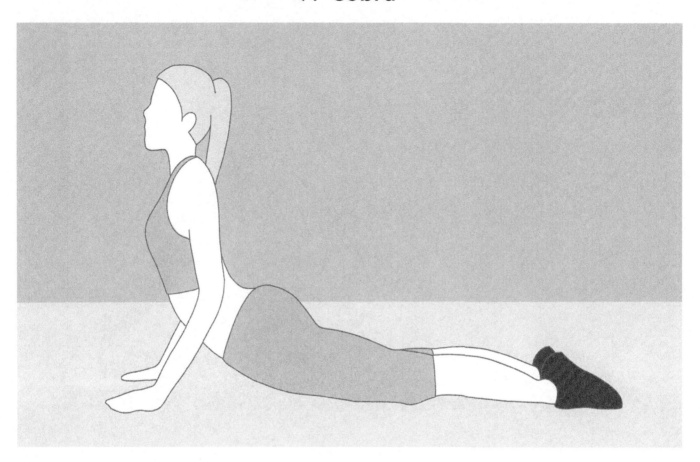

Sets x Repetitions: 2x30"

Muscles targeted: Abs, Arms, Shoulders

Equipment needed: Mat

Directions:

- Lie on your stomach and spread your legs behind you.

- Place your hands shoulder-width apart.

- With palms resting on the floor, slowly lift your upper body up, until you are positioned as in the image.

- Focus on feeling a stretch in both your chest and back muscles.

- Hold the position for 30 seconds.

- Repeat 2 times.

1. Back Pull

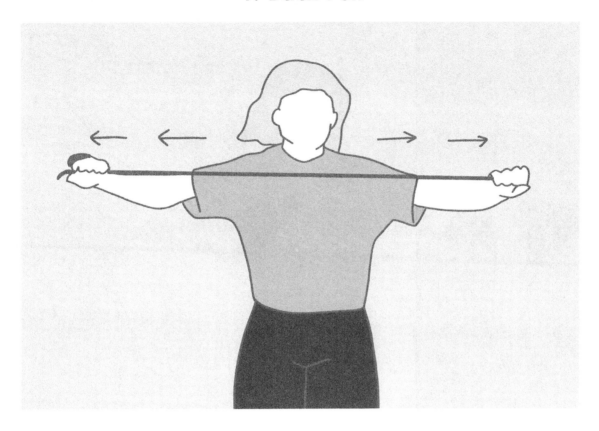

Sets x Repetitions: 3x8

Muscles targeted: Upper back, Shoulders

Equipment needed: Resistance band

Directions:

- Take both ends of the resistance band in your hands. As in the figure, your elbows should be slightly bent in front of your chest. If the band you have is too long, fold it in half.

- Pull the hands close to each other as you inhale.

- Push both arms outward, trying to straighten them as much as possible, focusing on contracting your upper back muscles.

- Return to the starting position and repeat 7 more times.

- Rest for 60 seconds, then repeat two more times.

2. Bent-Over Row

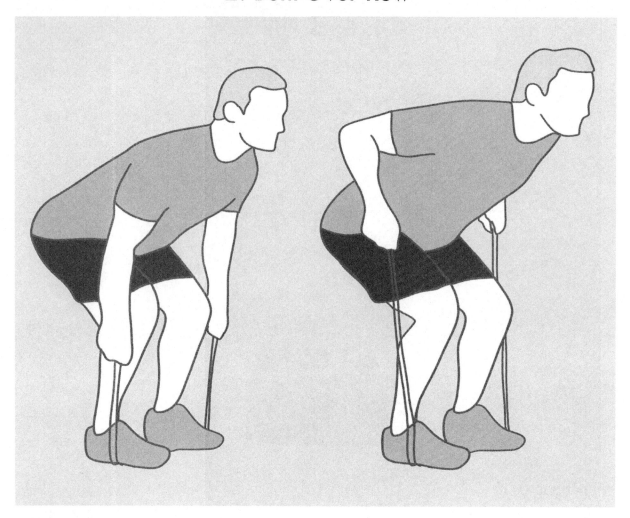

Sets x Repetitions: 3x8

Muscles targeted: Back

Equipment needed: Resistance band

Directions:

- Step on the resistance band and grab both ends, then bend your knees as in the figure above.

- Bend your torso forward until your upper body is almost parallel to the floor, tightening your core to protect your lower back from injuries.

- Pull the band upward slowly as you exhale. Your shoulder blades should be drawing closer together, and your elbows should be close to the body and facing the ceiling.

- Return to the starting position, then repeat the exercise 7 times for 2 more sets.

3. Bicep Curl

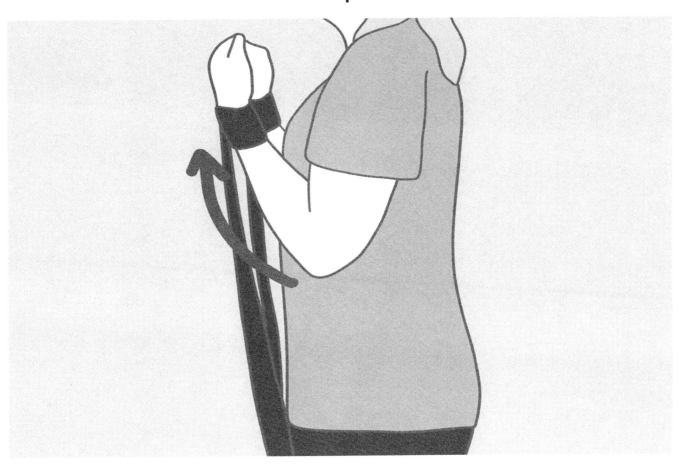

Sets x Repetitions: 3x12

Muscles targeted: Biceps

Equipment needed: Resistance band

Directions:

- Step with your feet on the center of the resistance band.

- Take both ends in your palms and grip them tightly. Your arms should be resting close to the body.

- Raise your arms in front of you up to your chest, trying to squeeze the biceps. Make sure your elbows always are next to the body for the whole range of motion.

- Hold the position for 1 second, then return to the starting position.

- Repeat the movement 11 times more for a total of 3 sets.

4. Lateral Raise

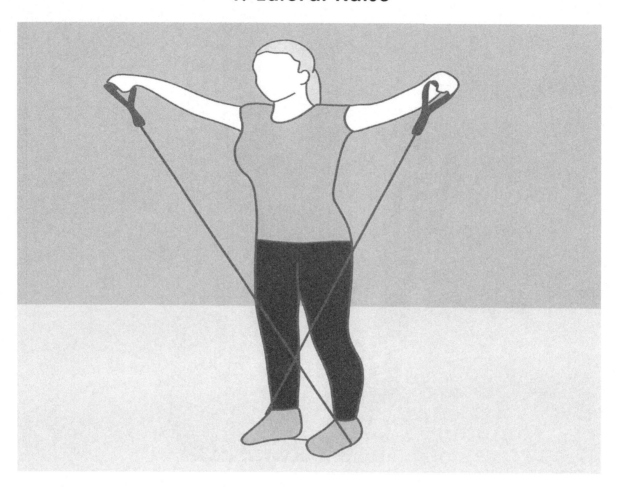

Sets x Repetitions: 3x10

Muscles targeted: Shoulders

Equipment needed: Resistance band

Directions:

- Step in the middle of your resistance band with both feet flat on the floor while standing.

- Take both handles of your band in your hands. You can grab the handles the standard way or as in the figure above (intertwined).

- Raise both arms to the side up to shoulder height so they are parallel to the floor.

- Slowly lower your arms until they form a 90° angle to the floor.

- Repeat the movement 9 more times for a total of 3 sets.

5. Squat With band

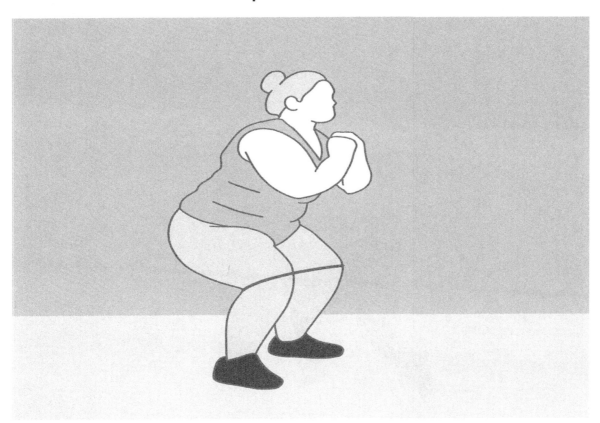

Sets x Repetitions: 3x8

Muscles targeted: Legs, Glutes, Abductors

Equipment needed: Resistance band

Directions:

- Stand straight with legs shoulder-width apart (feet slightly pointing outwards) and the resistance band placed around your legs, a few inches above the knees.

- Open the legs a bit more until you feel the resistance band is working against you, but you still can manage it.

- Engage your abs and slowly start to sit back. Make sure to keep your chest up, abs engaged and back straight. Of course, you want to sit down as much as you are comfortable to.

- Then, stand back up by pushing through the heels of your feet.

- Repeat the movement 8 times total. Rest for 1 minute, then repeat two more times.

6. Chest Press

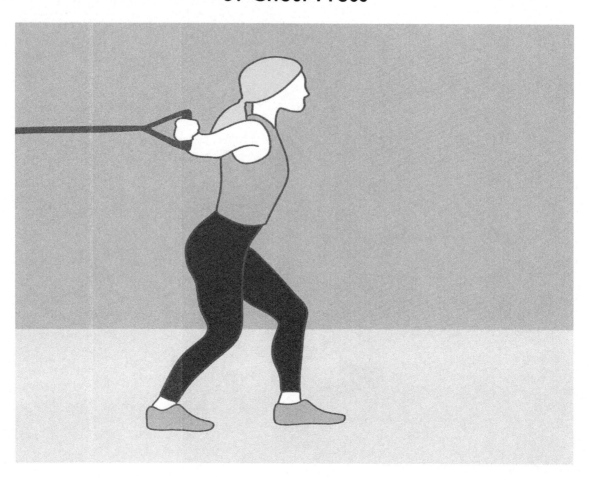

Sets x Repetitions: 3x8

Muscles targeted: Chest, Shoulders

Equipment needed: Resistance band

Directions:

- Stand straight with one leg in front of you and the other slightly behind your body for better stability.

- Hold both ends of the resistance band behind your shoulders while keeping the elbows slightly bent (palms facing each other).

- Bring the ends of the elastic band forward by extending your arms, and let the palms touch in front of your chest. Then, slowly return to the starting position (allowing your elbows to bend again).

- Repeat the movement 8 times total. Rest 60 seconds, then repeat two more times.

7. Leg Press with Band

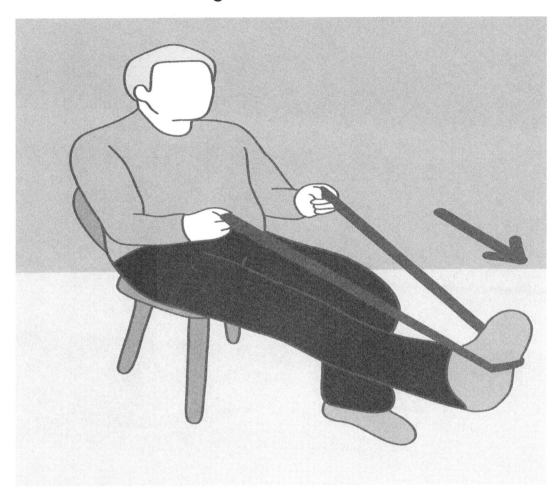

Sets x Repetitions: 3x10

Muscles targeted: Quads

Equipment needed: Resistance band

Directions:

- Sit on a chair with your back straight.

- Keep both ends of the resistance band in your hands.

- While keeping the leg foot on the ground, place the right one in the middle of the band.

- While holding both ends of the band, straighten your right leg in front of you. Then, return to the starting position (right knee bent).

- Repeat the movement 9 times. Then, switch legs and repeat for a total of 3 sets per leg.

BOSU/EXERCISE BALL WORKOUT
1. Heel Digs on Bosu

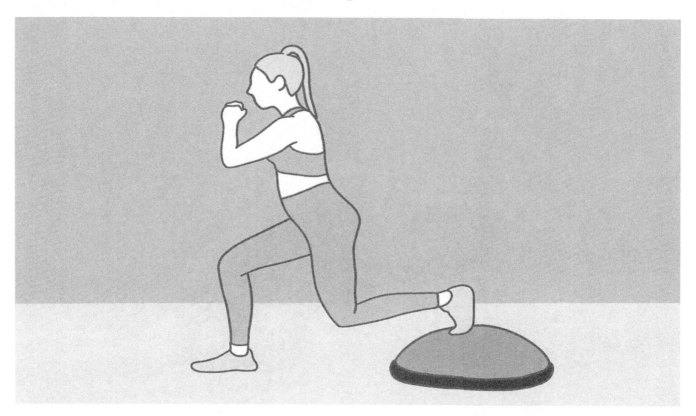

Sets x Repetitions: 3x8

Muscles targeted: Legs, Glutes

Equipment needed: Bosu

Directions:

- Stand in front of the bosu and rest the tip of your left foot on it. Make sure to put your right foot far enough from your body to ensure perfect execution.

- With the finger interlaced for better stability, slowly lower your right leg and let your left leg follow. Make sure your back stays straight during the movement. The range of motion stops when your left knee is a few inches from the floor.

- Slowly come back up, then repeat the movement 7 times more.

- Do the same for the other leg, then repeat the exercise for a total of 3 sets per leg,

2. Glute Bridge on Bosu

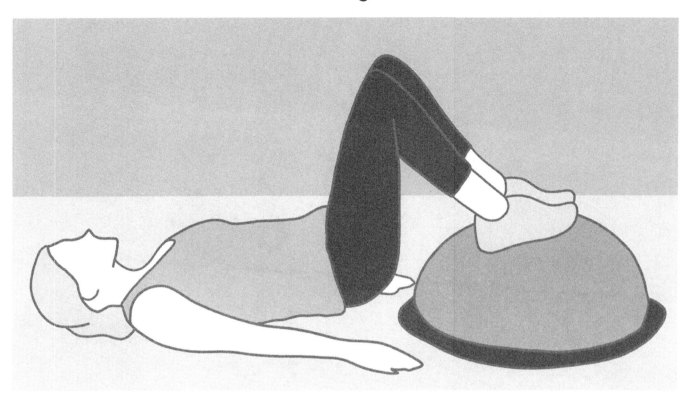

Sets x Repetitions: 3x30"

Muscles targeted: Abs, Glutes

Equipment needed: Bosu

Directions:

- Lie down on a mat with the soles of your feet on the bosu.

- Keep your arms along your sides and palms wide open on the floor for better stability.

- Contracts your glutes and lifts your hips as much as possible.

- Hold this position for 30 seconds, then return to the starting position.

- Rest for 30 seconds, then repeat for two more sets.

3. Basic Stance on Bosu

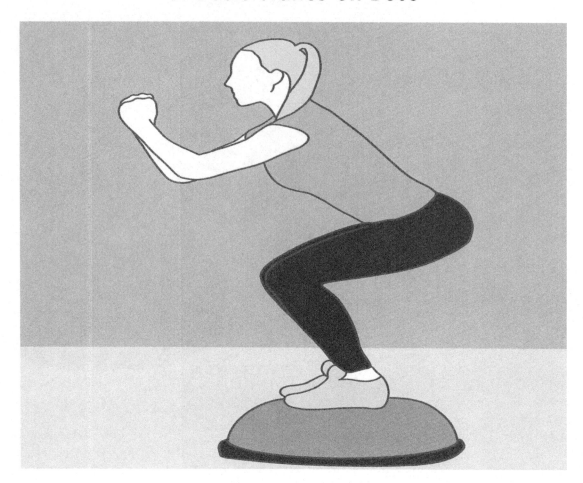

Sets x Repetitions: 3x30" or 3x60"

Muscles targeted: Abs, Legs, Glutes

Equipment needed: Bosu

Directions:

- Step onto the bosu with feet open wide. You might want a chair or something else to grab onto since this exercise can be tricky for beginners.

- Standing still will cause your feet to move and your torso to contract to find balance. You can increase the difficulty by letting go of the chair, extending your arms upwards, or closing your eyes.

- Bend your knees slightly as if performing a squat.

- Hold the position for 30 to 60 seconds.

- Rest for 60 seconds, then repeat for two more sets.

4. Compressions on Bosu

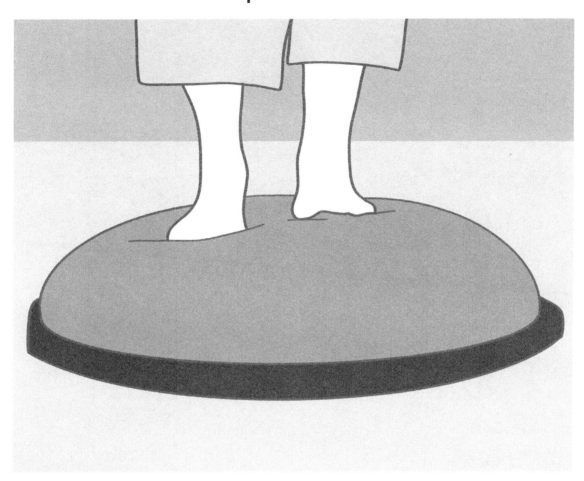

Sets x Repetitions: 2x45"

Muscles targeted: Abs, Glutes

Equipment needed: Bosu

Directions:

- Step onto the bosu with feet close to each other. You might want a chair or something else to grab onto since this exercise can be tricky for beginners.

- Once you find your balance, start digging your feet through the bosu one after the other.

- Perform this exercise for 45 seconds.

- Rest for 60 seconds, then repeat one more time.

5. Bosu Squat

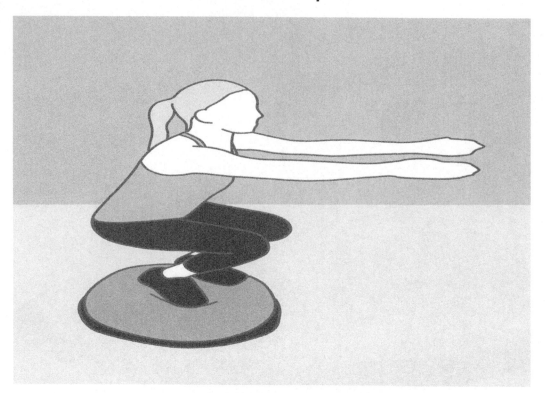

Sets x Repetitions: 3x8

Muscles targeted: Abs, Legs, Glutes

Equipment needed: Bosu

Directions:

- Step onto the bosu with feet open wide. You might want a chair or something else to grab onto since this exercise can be tricky for beginners.

- Squat down with your knees bent (pointing outward) as if sitting back on a chair, trying to go as low as you can.

- To help you keep balance, keep your back straight and your torso high, and extend your arms in front of you.

- Come back up, pushing mostly from the heels, not the tip of your feet. You may need to experiment with different foot positions to find one that allows you to retain your balance while squatting. Repeat the exercise 7 more times, for 3 sets total.

6. Kick Back on Bosu

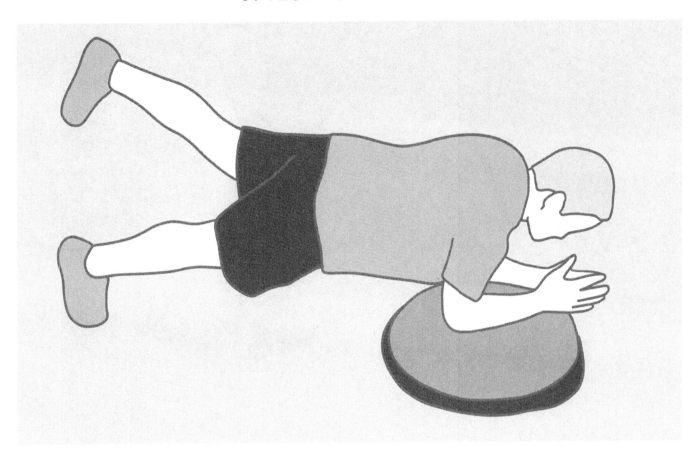

Sets x Repetitions: 3x10

Muscles targeted: Abs, Legs, Glutes

Equipment needed: Bosu

Directions:

- On all fours, place your knees on the mat and forearms on the bosu.

- Lift yourself up so that your body is horizontal.

- With the knee slightly bent. Lift the left leg back as much as you can while pressing the heel towards the ceiling. You should feel a nice contraction of the left glute when the heel gets in the highest position.

- Repeat the movement 9 more times.

- Do the same for the other leg, for a total of 3 sets per leg.

7. Crunch on Bosu

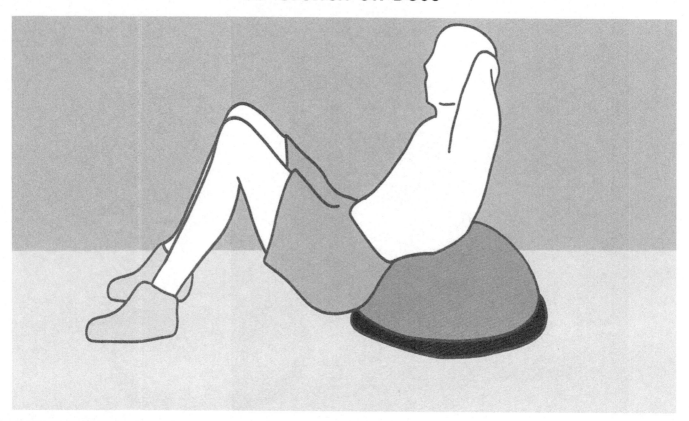

Sets x Repetitions: 3x15

Muscles targeted: Abs

Equipment needed: Bosu

Directions:

- Sit with your back on the bosu, your knees bent, and your feet flat on the floor.

- Interlace your fingers behind your head.

- While inhaling, roll back until you feel a stretch in your abs.

- Then, while exhaling, curl up, contracting your abs.

- Repeat the movement 14 times more.

- Rest 30 seconds, then repeat the exercise two more times.

1. Seated Bicep Curls

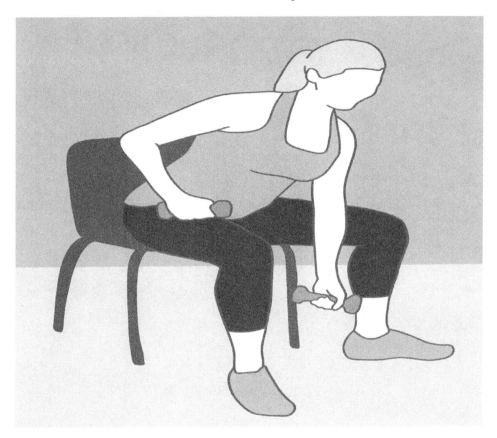

Sets x Repetitions: 2x7

Muscles targeted: Biceps

Equipment needed: Dumbell/Water bottle

Directions:

- Sit on a chair with your legs open wide and back leaned forward.

- Grab a dumbbell/water bottle and rest your elbow on your inner thigh as in the figure.

- Lift the weight toward you by contracting only the biceps muscle.

- Repeat the exercise 6 more times and then switch arms.

- Do 2 sets total per arm.

2. Hammer Curls

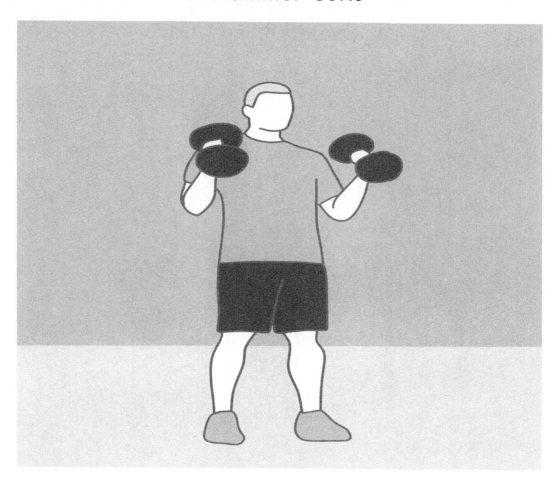

Sets x Repetitions: 2x7

Muscles targeted: Biceps

Equipment needed: Dumbell/Water bottle

Directions:

- Stand straight with legs shoulder-width apart.

- Hold a dumbbell in each hand with your palms facing inwards. Make sure to keep your hands in this position and your elbows tucked into your sides.

- Alternating between sides, lift the weight straight up to your shoulder. Actively squeeze your bicep muscle when you reach the top of the lift. Make sure to lower the weights slowly without swinging. Repeat the movement 6 more times per side.

- Rest for 60 seconds, then repeat the exercise one more time.

3. Single-Arm Overhead Triceps Extension

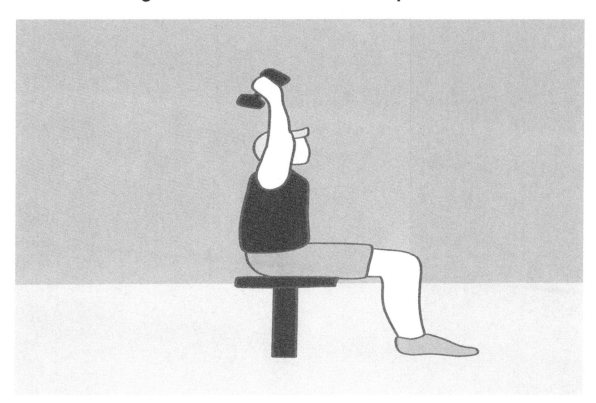

Sets x Repetitions: 2x7

Muscles targeted: Triceps

Equipment needed: Dumbell/Water bottle

Directions:

- Sit on a chair without a rest seat.

- Take a weight in one hand and extend your arm straight up to the sky.

- While keeping your back straight, lower the weight behind you, focusing on bending the elbow and keeping your upper arm and shoulder as stationary as possible. All the work must be done by your tricep muscle.

- Bring the weight as low as possible. Then, push the weight up using your tricep without moving your shoulder.

- Repeat the full movement 6 more times, then switch arms.

- Repeat the exercise one more time for both arms.

4. Skull Crusher

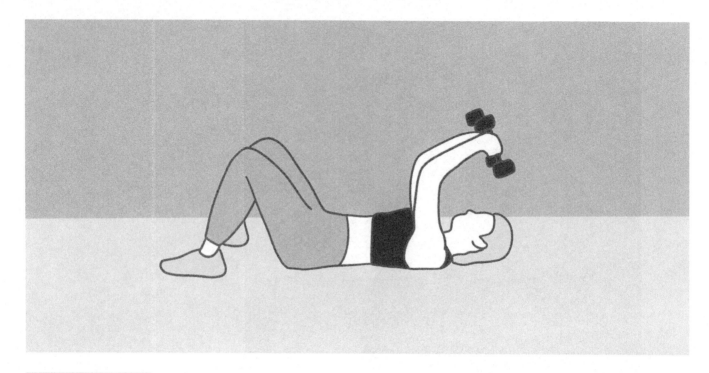

Sets x Repetitions: 2x7

Muscles targeted: Triceps

Equipment needed: Dumbell/Water bottle

Directions:

- Lie down on a mat with your knees slightly bent for better stability.

- Hold a weight in both hands, palms facing each other.

- Slowly lower both weights towards your head, focusing on keeping the elbows closed so that the triceps work the best. Again, the shoulders should stay still; like in the previous exercise, the triceps muscles do all the work.

- Push the weight up again, focusing on contracting the triceps.

- Repeat the movement 6 more times.

- Rest for 60 seconds, then repeat the exercise one more time.

5. Tricep Kickbacks

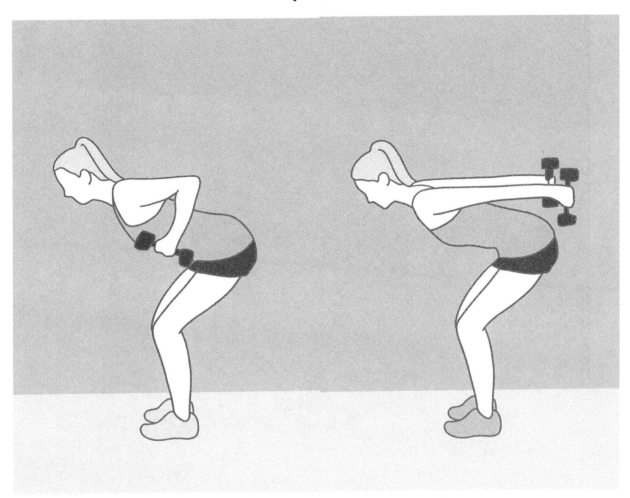

Sets x Repetitions: 10 minutes

Muscles targeted: arm, leg and shoulder

Equipment needed: dumbbell

Directions:

- Stand with a weight in both hands, and your feet close a few inches to each other.

- Lean your torso forward and flex your legs a little bit, keeping the back straight.

- With your arms at 90 degrees, push the dumbbell backward by extending your arm. Again, the shoulders should stay still; like in the previous exercise, the triceps muscles do all the work.

- Repeat the movement 9 more times. Rest 60 seconds, then repeat the exercise one more time.

6. Tricep Pulldown

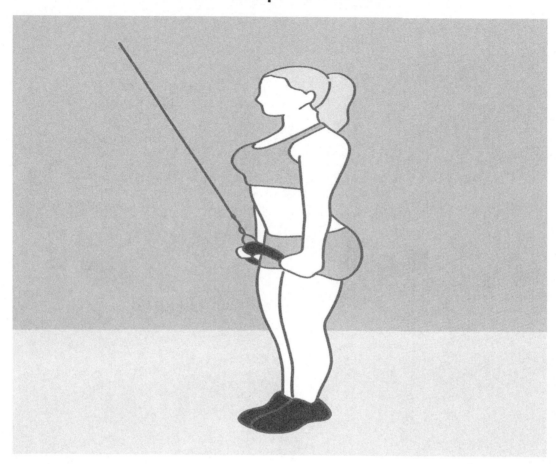

Sets x Repetitions: 2x10

Muscles targeted: Triceps

Equipment needed: Resistance band

Directions:

- Attach your resistance band to the top of a door or anything where it is securely tied and won't come loose.

- Pull down on the band with both hands simultaneously until your arms are fully extended. Then, slowly return them to your starting position. Ensure you maintain your posture throughout – Your back should be straight, knees slightly bent, and all the power must come from the triceps.

- Repeat the movement 9 more times.

- Rest 60 seconds, then repeat the exercise one more time.

COOLING-DOWN EXERCISES

1. Bear Hug

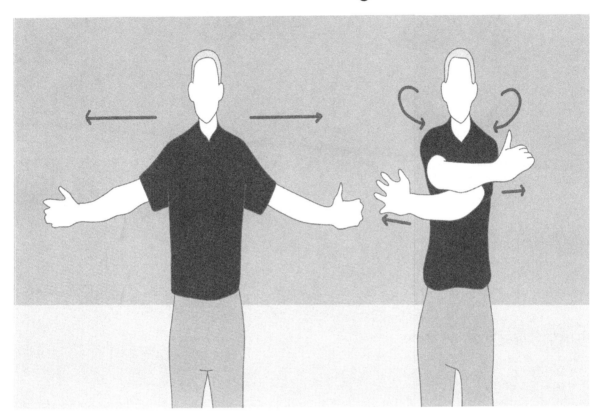

Targeted Area: Shoulders, Upper back

Difficulty: Easy

Directions:

- Stand with legs shoulder-width apart.

- Raise both arms straight on the sides (chest height)

- Hug yourself, trying to touch the opposite side of your back with both hands.

- Hold the stretched position for 2 seconds-

- Return to the starting position.

- Repeat the exercise 10 times.

2. Side-Lying Windmill Stretch

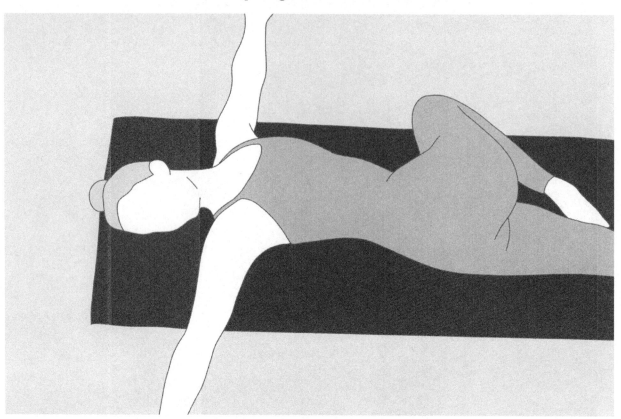

Targeted Area: Hip, thigh and groin

Difficulty: Medium

Directions:

- Lie on your left with your legs extended out in front of you.

- Cross your right leg over your left leg so that your right foot rests on the left leg.

- Put your left hand on your right knee and your right hand on the ground far from the body (for better stability).

- Rotate your torso to the right while your left hand pushes the right knee toward the floor.

- Twist until your feel a nice stretch (or your back is fully lying on the mat) and hold for 10-15 seconds.

- Repeat on the opposite side.

3. Calf Stretch

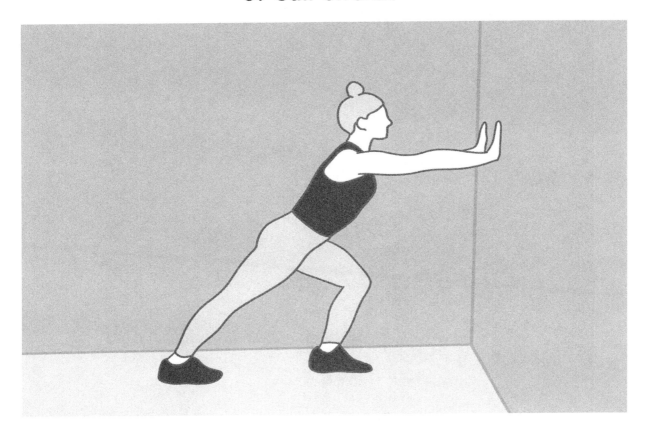

Targeted Area: Calf, Hamstring

Difficulty: Easy

Directions:

- Position yourself in front of a wall and rest both palms on it.

- Bring your front leg forward and bend it slightly.

- Stretch the back leg behind you as much as you can. You should feel a deep stretch in the calf.

- Hold the position for 30 seconds.

- Repeat the exercise for the other leg.

4. Knee Hug

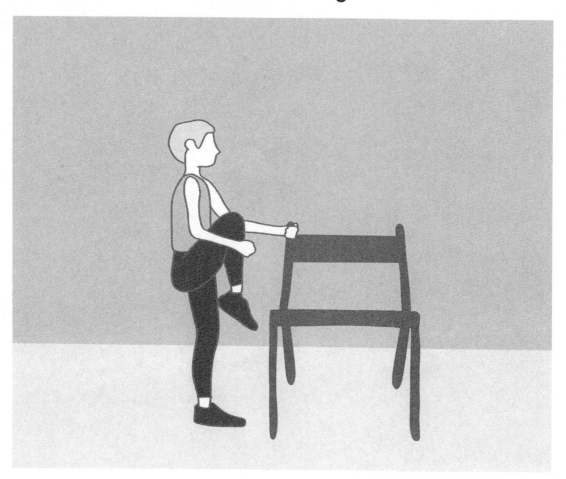

Targeted Area: Calf, Hamstring

Difficulty: Easy

Directions:

- Stand in front of a chair and grab the knee of your right leg with your right hand while holding onto the chair's back with the left hand for better stability

- Shift your body weight to your left leg.

- Pull the right knee as close to the chest as possible.

- Hold the position for 20 seconds, and then repeat the exercise for the other leg.

5. Cat-cow Stretch

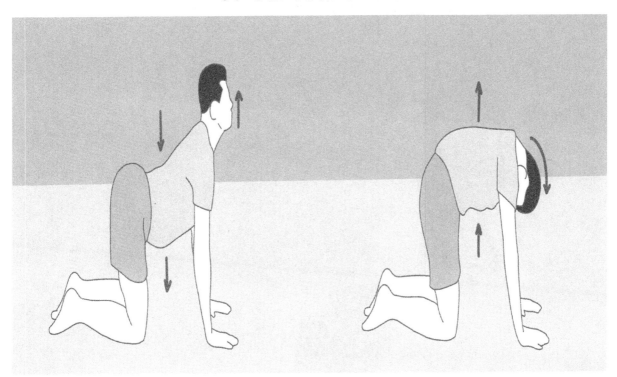

Targeted Area: Lower back, Upper back

Difficulty: Medium

Directions:

- Rest on all fours on the floor with your back neutral and parallel to the floor.

- Take a deep breath in and push your upper back toward the ceiling. Your lower back should be arched at this point.

- Rest in this position for 5 seconds.

- Slowly start exhaling while lowering your chin and contracting the abs. Your back should be curved as in the right photo now.

- Keep exhaling slowly while resting in this position for 5 seconds.

- Repeat the process 5 times.

6. Hamstring Stretch with Band

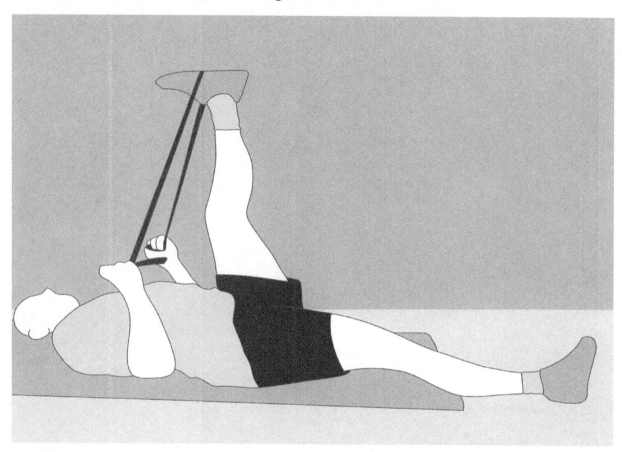

Targeted Area: Calf, Hamstring

Difficulty: Medium

Directions:

- Lie on your back on a mat.

- Place the strap around your left foot by bending the knee. Both hands should be on the strap.

- Straighten your left leg and lift it toward the ceiling, using the strap to control the intensity of the stretch.

- Rest in this position for 30 seconds.

- Repeat on the opposite side.

STAYING FIT AS YOU AGE

These 16 tips for staying fit as you age are the best I have recommended to my clients for years, and I have gotten positive feedback from them. I hope as you read and take the necessary actions, you will begin to see the result in no time.

1) Drink at least 2 liters of water daily. Water flushes toxins out of your cells and keeps them hydrated, which improves circulation, helps fight wrinkles, and keeps you looking younger too! That means no soda/energy drinks or anything that contains caffeine because it could worsen dehydration. Moreover, some side effects can be headaches, raised blood pressure, and irregular heartbeat. If the situation worsens, then death can occur...so try to avoid drinking too much or any caffeinated beverages. Do drink more water than usual for these exercises but make sure that you don't overdo it with water intake as well because if you do, then it won't benefit anyone... just remember -consult your doctor first before starting to drink lots of water.

2) Eat healthy, nutritious food daily. Avoid snacks high in sugar, sodium or saturated fat because these foods can lead to many health problems like weight gain, poor digestion, depression, diabetes and many more! If you consume too much-processed food, try switching to fresh fruit/vegetables, which contain vitamins & minerals that will benefit you greatly, so why not give them a chance? Make sure you don't overeat either because it is bad for your overall health if you do...but stick with mostly eating fruits/vegetables instead of anything else daily-it's worth it! You should eat healthy because if you don't, it will take a huge toll on your health.

3) Try to exercise at least 3 times a week for about 20 minutes each time. Exercise is very important after age 60+, and even though some people forget that, doctors say that seniors should still exercise at least 2-3 hours per week (as a beginner, of course). It's best to perform exercises slowly rather than trying something new or fast-paced, which can cause more injuries. Instead of helping in any way...just listen to your body and adjust accordingly whenever possible.

4) Don't smoke cigarettes or marijuana because they are not healthy for our overall health. If you do those things, your body will be in a worse condition than before, plus smoking is the leading cause of death in America. Every year, approximately 480,000 people die from cigarette smoking which costs our country millions of dollars because that money could have been spent on more important issues...and marijuana is also harmful to our health if we do it too much (but don't worry about occasional bong/joint use).

5) Eat foods high in vitamin C like oranges, tomato juice, or broccoli because they can help boost your immune system. When you are sick with a cold or flu, you need lots of rest and staying warm at home—not just for healing but so that you don't spread the infection to others. Your immune system can also be helped with a healthy diet of fruits, vegetables and whole grains to keep your energy up for a longer time throughout the day.

6) Do light daily exercise at home if you want an active life! Even just doing basic things like taking the stairs instead of elevators or escalators and walking around more often rather than sitting all day is beneficial for your body because those simple exercises can burn calories as well. So why not try them out? It will boost your endurance and strength but use common sense as always when doing strenuous exercises (for example, don't lift too much weight).

7) If you have problems sleeping at night, try doing light exercises before bed. Some people are so stressed that they can't get proper rest during the night because of constant nagging health issues or even insomnia. Exercise helps calm your mind and relax properly before heading off to sleep. Of course, it's always best to find a simple routine that works for you daily but be careful not to overdo it during nighttime workouts (in case you need 3 hours of sleep).

8) Keep your body temperature stable by wearing comfortable clothes. Remember it's important not to wear anything too warm or too cool because it will cause many health problems like skin rashes, eczema, diabetes, varicose veins and so forth. Also, get enough sleep at night (approximately 7 hours) if you want your body temperature balanced properly.

9) Have fun doing exercises even though they are simple home workouts! After all, exercise isn't just about what you do but how you feel when doing it. If you enjoy exercising, that matters most because that is a sign of true happiness...or if you don't enjoy it, then consider changing your routine by mixing exercises up or stopping altogether to try something new until you find one that suits you perfectly.

10) Do some light stretching before you begin doing home exercises. Simple yoga postures are always a great way to start any workout routine but even just taking deep breaths and walking around is good before going nuts with the weights...if you want to live an active lifestyle, try it out!

11) If you have joint problems or other injuries, you should always listen to your doctor if he says not to exercise. However, even if you can't do strenuous running, plenty of exercises don't involve those things. So be cautious about taking risks when exercising (and, most importantly, listen to your body).

12) Be sure to listen to your mind and body when exercising. If you feel pain or have problems, you must stop immediately.

13) To get rid of fat, ensure you do some aerobics a few times a week and remember to eat healthy food. Try to avoid eating fatty foods or drinking soda because it is unhealthy for your body as well... also be sure to get about 30 minutes of sunlight outdoors every day if you want good health!

14) The essential thing to remember is that when aging, it is also normal for your body to change and undergo many different changes. So don't let society's views of how you should look at a certain age affect how you are...instead just be yourself and live each day happily because if you can do that, you will always stay young at heart!

15) When exercising as a senior, don't overdo it. Firstly, just check with your doctor. As long as your knees are in good shape or else they have been properly rehabilitated after any kind of surgery, plenty of exercises you can do at home that will help strengthen your joints. There are many types of simple exercises for seniors, which is why it's best to experiment by trying something new until you find something that works for your individual needs...but remember to always be cautious about what you are doing, especially when exercising on your own.

16) Even something as simple as weight training at home can put years back onto your body if done correctly. Still, if not, it might actually have a negative effect by weakening muscles and joints...to avoid injuries from weights at home, be sure to listen to your body and also try doing different exercises because no two person's bodies are alike.

MYTHS AND MISCONCEPTIONS

There are various myths and misconceptions about old age. I'll review some of the most common ones that keep older people from participating in physical activities.

MYTH #1: AS YOU BECOME OLDER, YOU LOSE YOUR ABILITY TO EXERCISE.

The more involved you are, on the other hand, the greater your tolerance for physical exertion and the more you can accomplish during the day. Your activity tolerance diminishes when you stop doing any type of physical activity. According to a University of Georgia study, subjects who exercised for 20 minutes three times a week for six weeks experienced a 65 percent reduction in weariness (Puetz et al., 2008).

According to a study, participation in sports and exercise has been shown to boost general physical activity and energy levels. In addition, maintaining an active lifestyle will assist you in lowering your resting heart rate, increasing your blood pressure, and even increasing your metabolic rate.

Myth No. 2: People over 60 are too old to exercise.

Fauja Singh is the world's oldest marathon runner, finishing his last race in 2013 at 101. However, he has demonstrated that age is nothing more than a number that does not influence one's capacity to exercise. In 2015, 49 percent of marathon runners in the United States were classified as "masters," indicating they were 40 years old or older. In addition, 200 adults aged 60 and over were evaluated in a randomized controlled trial about home fitness programs. Improvements in balance and impairment scores were measured after the project. None of the subjects reported any negative health impacts (Evans, 2017).

Anyone (regardless of age) can stimulate their heart and lungs to raise their heart and breathing rate, according to Dr. Thomas Boyden, MS, program director of preventive cardiology at SHMG Cardiovascular Medicine in Grand Rapids, Michigan. As a result, the circulatory and respiratory systems are stimulated, reducing the risk of cardiovascular disorders like heart attacks and strokes and the danger of cancer (Citroner, 2019).

Myth #3: What's the point of exercising if I'm already old?

Exercise lowers the risk of Alzheimer's disease and dementia, heart disease, diabetes, several malignancies, high blood pressure, and obesity. Exercise can have the same influence on one's mood at 70 or 80 as it did when they were 20 or 30. This myth is mainly about complacency, a human inclination to stay put because any type of change requires some work, no matter how beneficial. If you're having trouble getting started, remind yourself of the benefits that will come once you begin any type of physical activity.

Myth #4: Exercising makes me more likely to fall and break my bones.

Contrary to popular belief, regular exercise improves balance and minimizes the chance of falling by improving strength and endurance. Over 200 million individuals worldwide suffer from osteoporosis, producing brittle, fragile, and easily shattered bones. Osteoporosis affects 30% of postmenopausal women, and one in every six women will break their hip at some point in their lives. As you get older, there are techniques to strengthen your bones. Most of these therapies would also improve physical health and life expectancy. These approaches necessitate you getting up and moving (5 Ways to Strengthen Older Bones, 2021).

MYTH #5: I USED TO BE AN ATHLETE. I DON'T THINK I'M CAPABLE OF DOING IT ALL OVER AGAIN.

Because of changes in hormones, physiology, metabolism, bone density, body composition, and muscle mass, overall strength and efficiency levels will definitely decline with age. However, physical activity does not rule out the possibility of acquiring a sense of success or improving your health. Setting realistic lifestyle goals for your age group is crucial. Remember that a sedentary lifestyle has a considerably greater impact on physical performance than biological aging.

The good news is that athletes had a lower age-related drop-in maximum heart rate than non-athletes. The same benefits are anticipated to accrue to older persons who engage in vigorous fitness training as their younger counterparts.

MYTH #6: OH, THIS IS TOO DIFFICULT! I'M TOO OLD TO WORK OUT!

It's important to remember that it's never too late to start exercising and getting in better shape! Adults who become physically and cognitively active later in life show more profound improvements than younger people. You won't get the same sports injuries as many everyday exercisers later in life if you've never exercised previously or haven't done so in a long time. In other words, you won't have to worry about past injuries reoccurring and causing discomfort. Begin with easy routines and progress from there (Robinson et al., 2020).

Regardless of your level of exercise in your youth, Dr. Richard J. Hodes, director of the NIH National Institute of Aging, says it's crucial to get started and stay active. We must recognize the importance of people remaining self-sufficient for as long as possible. Seniors can keep their physical function by exercising and engaging in greater physical activity in their everyday lives, which is necessary for them to perform the activities they wish to do.

MYTH #7: BECAUSE I'M DISABLED, I'M NOT ALLOWED TO EXERCISE!

Being challenged comes with its own set of problems. If you are confined to a chair, you confront particular obstacles. Lifting modest weights, stretching, and doing chair aerobics, chair yoga, and chair tai chi can help you increase your range of motion, muscular tone and endurance, and cardiovascular health. Many pools are wheelchair accessible, and adaptive fitness programs for wheelchair sports such as basketball are also provided. People with disabilities can follow the same requirements as healthy individuals or do as much as possible to avoid being inactive, according to the 2008 Physical Activity Guidelines.

MYTH #8: I'M TOO FRAIL TO EXERCISE.

Moving about will ease discomfort while also boosting your strength and self-esteem. Unfortunately, many senior citizens discover that regular exercise slows and enhances the decline of strength and stamina as they age. The idea is to start cautiously and gradually increase the number of activities as you gain strength. In the 1970s, several investigations of stable older individuals indicated that resilience, endurance, and flexibility declined considerably after age 55. For example, according to the Framingham Disability Report, 62% of women aged 75 to 85 had difficulty bending or bowing down, 66% couldn't lift more than 10 pounds, and 42% couldn't stand for more than 15 minutes. Once upon a time, these decreases were considered an unavoidable aspect of aging. However, a seminal study released in 1994 by Harvard and Tufts researchers indicated that many functional deficits might be restored, particularly in the frailest and oldest women (Exercise after Age 70, 2019).

According to popular thinking, the more active you are, the healthier your life will be (Exercise after Age 70, 2019).

MUSCLE RECOVERY

Regular exercise is key to a healthy, strong body and peak physical fitness. However, if you want to get the most out of your regular workout, that is, getting into your desired body shape while avoiding injuries, you will need to allow your muscles adequate time to recover.

If you think resting from working out for a day will always set you back, think again. After working out, you must give your body sufficient breaks before exercising again to allow it to recover from the previous workout.

Most train people tend to overlook the notion that exercise is stress. Yes, it is. But wait..., did this statement confuse you? Don't get confused. This is not the same type of stress I am talking about. This is good stress. Exercise stresses your muscles which provides long-lasting benefits in the end.

Any intense exercise creates fatigue, micro-traumas, and tears in your muscles. Muscle soreness and pain are the most common symptoms of this effect.

After exercise, lactic acid accumulates within your body cells. There is scientific evidence that lactic acid impairs the electrical stimulus required for muscle contraction when it builds up in your muscles. It also impairs your body's ability to generate ATP. This essential molecule plays a big role in repeated muscle contraction.

None of the above sounds beneficial, right? However, it is until you factor in the recovery period that's when you will enjoy the fruits of your workout efforts. First, we must create a healing environment for these micro-traumas and tears to repair. Through recovery, your body will eliminate lactic acid from your muscles and restore its capacity to produce ATP.

WAYS IN WHICH OUR MUSCLES RECOVER

The six elements of muscle recovery are stretching, rest, nutrition, hydration, sleep, and massage. Let's look at each element in detail.

1. STRETCHING

Stretching is an important aspect of exercise; that's why it is recommended that you include it in your workout routine. But many people tend to neglect it. Dynamic stretching before a workout keeps your body open, giving your muscles space and flexibility to complete the moves safely and through a full range of motion. This helps reduce the risks of injury, muscle soreness, and tears. On the other hand, stretching after a workout helps heal your muscles and reduce DOMS.

2. REST DAYS

If you are following a workout program, you will always hear people remind you about your workout days and how you need to exercise regularly. But you will never hear anyone talk about rest.

You must include rest days in your workout routine to achieve your training goals and adhere to them. They help your body repair and recover faster. As discussed earlier, the process of muscle building takes 2-4 days. And while most experts recommend full-body strength training for 2-3 non-consecutive days per week, this may vary from person to person. The news is that there is a way your body communicates when it needs rest.

SIGNS THAT YOU NEED REST

If you have any of the following signs, know that your body needs rest, and it will help if you plan for a rest day:

- Decreased performance. If you stop seeing progress, or you start having difficulty carrying out your exercises, take a rest day.

- Lack of sleep. If you can't sleep for at least 7-8 hours every night, take some rest from your workout.

- Sore muscles. Although it is common and normal to feel sore after your workout, it shouldn't go for a prolonged period. If the soreness is persistent, you need to take action. It is a sign that your muscles have yet to recover from the previous workouts and need some time.

- Pain. Consistent muscle and joint pain might be a sign of injuries from overuse.

- Muscle fatigue. You need to rest if you feel extremely exhausted.

3.   NUTRITION

Both exercise and diet contribute in equal proportion to the fitness equation. After a workout, protein intake is key as it helps with refueling and recovery of your muscles. At this point, you already know that muscle contraction from consistent training causes micro-trauma and tears to your body muscles. To repair and rebuild these muscles, you will need amino acids. This means you must consume protein to help supply your muscles with the amino acid.

By now, you're also aware that your body uses glycogen to fuel your workouts, and by the time you're done, your glycogen stores will have depleted. So to replenish your glycogen stores, you will also need to consume some carbs.

4.   HYDRATION

This may cause dehydration which may lower your performance. Therefore, you are advised to drink plenty of water before, during, and after the workout to keep your body hydrated.

The usual recommendation is to ensure that you drink at least 8 glasses or 2 liters of water every day. Electrolyte water can be a good option because besides keeping your body hydrated, it also supplies your body with important electrolytes like calcium, potassium, and magnesium, which also play a role in muscle recovery.

5.   SLEEP

There are two major stages of sleep: Rapid Eye Movement (REM) and Non-Rapid Eye Movement (Non-REM). Therefore, to understand the effect of sleep on muscle recovery, you must understand what happens in these two sleep phases.

RAPID EYE MOVEMENT (REM) SLEEP

This phase of sleep accounts for about 25% of your total sleep. It occurs in cycles of about 1.5 – 2 hours throughout the night. REM sleep dominates the latter half of your sleeping time. It provides your brain with energy that supports it during waking hours. It also restores your mind.

NON-REM SLEEP

This is the most important phase in muscle recovery. It is where deep sleep happens. That's why it is sometimes known as the slow-wave or deep sleep phase. It accounts for about 40% of your total sleep. During this phase, your blood pressure decreases, and your breathing becomes slower and deeper.

At this time, very few activities are going on in your brain because it is resting. As a result, the blood supply to your muscles increases, delivering extra amounts of oxygen and nutrients to your muscles. This enhances faster recovery and muscle growth.

Another important thing during this sleep phase is the secretion of growth hormones. As your body enters this phase, your pituitary glands release a shot of growth hormones that stimulate tissue growth and muscle repair. Failing to get enough sleep during the night can result in a sharp decline in the secretion of growth hormones.

Research indicates that deficiency of growth hormones is associated with muscle mass loss and reduced exercise capacity.

In summary, sleep enhances muscle recovery in two ways: protein synthesis and growth hormone secretion. So, if you want to increase muscle mass and recover faster from your previous workouts.

6.   MASSAGE

Massage your muscles after training. Massaging the worked muscles helps relieve the lactic acids that build up in the areas. This enhances faster recovery.

4-WEEK PLAN

WEEK 1

Day	Workout	Sets
Monday	Flexibility + Core-Focused	1
Wednesday	Balance + Sitting	1
Friday	Bosu Ball	2

WEEK 2

Day	Workout	Sets
Monday	Sitting + Standing	1
Tuesday	Arm Strength + Resistance Bands	1
Thursday	Flexibility + Balance	1
Friday	Core-Focused	2

WEEK 3

Day	Workout	Sets
Monday	Flexibility + Bosu Ball	1
Tuesday	Standing	2
Thursday	Arm Strength + Resistance Bands	1
Friday	Core-Focused	2

Day	Workout	Sets
Monday	Flexibility + Sitting	1
Tuesday	Bosu Ball + Core-Focused	1
Thursday	Arm Strength + Resistance Bands	1
Friday	Flexibility	2
Sunday	Core-Focused + Standing	1

INDEX

T

W

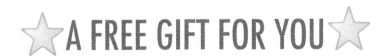 A FREE GIFT FOR YOU

Get the audio version for free and listen to the exercises nar-
rated by 65-year old Michael (my dad :D)

DOWNLOAD THE AUDIO VERSION FOR FREE

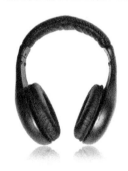

BENEFITS OF LISTENING TO THE AUDIO VERSION
- You don't have to keep the book open!
- You will feel in good company
- It keeps you more motivated

SCAN THE QR CODE INSIDE THE BOOK TO DOWNLOAD IT FOR FREE!

.

SCAN THE QR CODE BELOW TO ACCESS THE AUDIO FILES

SCAN ME

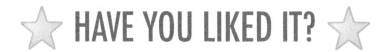

⭐ HAVE YOU LIKED IT? ⭐

To provide the best quality cases to customers, I would love to hear your thoughts and opinions on this collection.

TO DO SO, I WOULD ENCOURAGE YOU TO

LEAVE A HONEST REVIEW ON AMAZON.

Your comment will ultimately aid me in continually improving my current and future books. I genuinely hope that your experience with my product was positive and memorable!

SCAN ME

THANK YOU IN ADVANCE FOR YOUR VALUABLE FEEDBACK

THIS WILL HELP ME A LOT AS A SELF-PUBLISHED AUTHOR!

Printed in Great Britain
by Amazon

29323018R00057